# Mental health and well-being in later life

# Mental health and well-being in later life

*Edited by Mima Cattan*

 Open University Press

Open University Press
McGraw-Hill Education
McGraw-Hill House
Shoppenhangers Road
Maidenhead
Berkshire
England
SL6 2QL

email: enquiries@openup.co.uk
world wide web: www.openup.co.uk

and Two Penn Plaza, New York, NY 10121-2289, USA

First published 2009

A catalogue record of this book is available from the British Library

ISBN-13: 978-0-33-5228928 (pb) 978-0-33-5228911 (hb)
ISBN-10: 0-33-522892-5 (pb) 0-33-522891-7 (hb)

Typeset by Kerrypress, Luton, Bedfordshire
Printed and bound in the UK by Bell and Bain Ltd., Glasgow

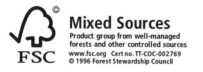

**Mixed Sources**
Product group from well-managed
forests and other controlled sources
www.fsc.org   Cert no. TT-COC-002769
© 1996 Forest Stewardship Council

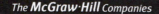

*The McGraw-Hill Companies*

# Contents

# List of tables, figures and boxes

## Figures

## Tables

## Boxes

# List of contributors

*Liz Aitchison* is a freelance Research Associate with the Faculty of Health and Social Care Sciences, Kingston University, and St George's, University of London. She also works with voluntary organizations supporting them in strategic development. With a background in social work followed by senior management in the voluntary sector, she has a special interest in well-being and ageing, and has been involved in a number of research studies in this field.

*Mima Cattan* is Reader in Health Promotion, Healthy Ageing, and Co-Director of the Centre for Health Promotion Research at Leeds Metropolitan University. She has a background in health promotion where she was involved in a range of mental health promotion and older people initiatives. Her PhD from the University of Newcastle focused on health promotion, and social isolation and loneliness among older people. Her main research interests relate to healthy ageing and mental health promotion, including transport and well-being in later life, quality of life and access to services among frail older people, and the concepts of health, well-being and ageing among older migrants. She is a co-editor with Sylvia Tilford of *Mental Health Promotion: A Lifespan Approach.*

*Angela Clow* is Professor of Psychophysiology at the University of Westminster. She trained in neuropharmacology, physiology and psychology, and likes to work at the interface of these disciplines. For her PhD (Institute of Psychiatry, London), she investigated the function of brain dopamine receptors and during her post-doctoral studies she developed an interest in the biochemistry of stress. She is a founder member of the Psychophysiology and Stress Research Group (PSRG) at the University of Westminster. Her current research investigates the physiological pathways by which stress and well-being can affect health and in particular the daily patterns of cortisol secretion. She has published over 91 full-length peer-reviewed papers, two books, and 25 book chapters or reviews.

*Denise Forte* is Principal Lecturer, Gerontology, in the Faculty of Health and Social Care Sciences, Kingston University, and St George's, University of London. She has extensive experience of working with older people in hospital and residential care settings in the UK and Australia, and maintains an interest in all aspects of ageing and how they are experienced by older people. She has developed a particular interest in relationships and sexuality in older age, on which she has written a number of papers. She also has a keen interest in ways in which older people engage in decisions about their own health and social care.

*Steve Iliffe* is Professor of Primary Care for Older People at University College London. He has worked in inner-city general practice for 30 years and has developed a research portfolio on health promotion in later life and on dementia care in the community. A member of the editorial boards of *Primary Health Care Research & Development*, *Aging & Health*, the *International Journal of Geriatric Psychiatry* and the

*Journal of Dementia Care*, he is also Associate Director of the Dementia and Neurology Diseases Research Network (DeNDRoN). His books include *Depression in Later Life*, co-authored with Jill Manthorpe, and the award-winning *From General Practice to Primary Care: The Industrialisation of Family Medicine*.

*Jill Manthorpe* is Professor of Social Work at King's College London and Director of the Social Care Workforce Research Unit. She has a background in the voluntary sector and currently researches in the area of workforce studies, dementia, depression, safeguarding and risk. She has written extensively on the subjects of depression and dementia in later life, and her recent books include *Older Workers in Europe* (edited with Anthony Chiva) and *Psychosocial Interventions in Early Dementia* (edited with Esme Moniz-Cook). She has a long-standing interest in adult safeguarding policy and practice that is fostered by regular discussion with practitioners and older people's groups.

*Maureen Mickus* is a gerontologist and Associate Professor in the Department of Occupational Therapy at Western Michigan University. Dr Mickus' research has focused on mental health issues in later life, conducting studies in dementia, depression and tele-health as an avenue for service delivery. She has also led studies related to ageing policy in both community and institutional care settings.

*Suzanne Moffatt* is Senior Lecturer in the Sociology of Health at the Institute of Health & Society, University of Newcastle. She trained as a speech and language therapist before embarking on a post-doctoral research career in 1990. Since 2000, she has undertaken a number of studies which have focused on health, welfare and well-being among older people. Her current and long-term interests are in the health and well-being of older people, the impact of changes to the welfare state on older people, tackling health and social inequalities and applying research to policy and practice. She has carried out extensive research into the impact of welfare rights advice on people over state retirement age and ethnic minority elders, and has published widely on the subject.

*Tom Owen* is a qualified social worker, and worked for 12 years in community care before joining Help the Aged as Research Manager where his brief was to commission and manage a range of studies related to services for vulnerable older people. He is currently on secondment to the Centre for Home Care Studies at City University, London, as Deputy Director of the My Home Life Programme. He has published several articles and reports on end of life care and the health service needs of older people.

*Sylvia Tilford* is Visiting Professor in Health Promotion at Leeds Metropolitan University. Before working for over 20 years at Leeds Met in postgraduate training for health promotion, she worked in school and adult education. She has a special interest in international developments in health promotion. Her interest in mental health promotion has been long-standing and related activities have included teaching, the review and dissemination of the evidence base for mental promotion and involvement in community health promotion projects. She is a co-editor with Mima Cattan of *Mental Health Promotion: A Lifespan Approach* and co-author with Keith Tones of *Health Promotion, Effectiveness, Efficiency and Equity*.

*Gill Windle* is a gerontologist based at Bangor University, where she studied as a mature student to obtain her BSc, MSc and PhD in Psychology. She is currently the research development fellow for two thematic networks: OPAN (Older people and ageing research and development network) and NEURODEM (Neurodegenerative diseases and dementias). Previously Gill has worked on a number of projects addressing the wider determinants of quality of life in older age. She has been actively involved in policy development in Wales. Her current research interests include health, mental well-being and resilience, and examining the interplay between internal, psychological factors and external, social factors on well-being outcomes.

# Foreword

Reading this book has made it abundantly clear just how much we have devalued old age – in the UK in particular as well as in the West more generally. It is not that we have devalued all older people – far from it. We have people who are 'national treasures' – admired because they go hang-gliding at 80 or are studying for a PhD at 90. But we see old age as a nuisance and older people as no longer contributing, and our obsession with body image makes us less at home with the ageing process than we should be. Add into that a disastrous professional desire to categorize older people into 'mentally ill' or 'physically disabled', a desire to provide accommodation in silos only with people who have been categorized in similar ways, and one can see all too easily why older people may find living a normal life less than easy, as they get frailer.

There is undoubtedly discrimination against older people as well as a tendency to medicalize ageing, with doctors seeing older people as being far less well than they think they are. That is why a serious review, which these chapters provide, of what it means to experience mental well-being in older age is so important, and that is why one of the themes that emerges time and again out of these chapters is the need to be needed. It is not just older people who need to be needed. It is part of the human make-up. We are not solitary animals and we live better and thrive better in partnerships and groups. So the emphasis in this volume on relationships, on work and occupation, on being active in many ways, as contributing to well-being both mentally and physically provides very welcome reading, as does the book's emphasis on retaining choice and control over how one lives, with whom, and how much it costs, looking at how poverty limits choice and autonomy, which are enormously important.

This book has a great deal to teach us. It celebrates much of getting older, and in particular grandparenthood. In the words of one of the many older people who contributed: 'I feel as if I've achieved something ... I've used my time usefully and they are kind of like the end product.' There is a meaning to being older, a sense of contribution, of satisfaction, and delight in intergenerational relationships that is wholly positive, which sits alongside some of the things that make life hard.

This book's main contribution, however, is to say to us all that there is no single solution, no magic bullet, no instant cure, for the discomforts and illnesses of older age – not all aspects of ageing are comfortable. But it also tells us that it is within our control to do something about much of these, that older people's mental well-being could be vastly improved, and that public policy and private attitudes need to change. I hope that the book is as influential as it deserves to be.

Baroness Julia Neuberger
Former Chief Executive of the King's Fund and author of *Not Dead Yet*

# Preface

Having worked with older people in a range of settings, taught undergraduate and postgraduate modules on mental health promotion and health promotion, and older people, and having been involved in research on promoting health in later life for many years, this book seemed the obvious text to write. However, this wasn't the only reason. It seemed that when it came to mental health (promotion) and older people, most texts focused on dementia or mental illness generally rather than on positive mental health and the factors involved in promoting well-being. This was rather strange, because when you talk to older people about their mental well-being, they usually raise issues such as relationships, social isolation, resources, pensions, housing, transport and mobility. They also frequently talk about ageism, being patronized and ignored and the stigma of being old as affecting their mental health. Finally, they point out that not all older people are the same, just as with younger people, they are not identical in their personalities, needs, desires, experiences, and so on. In this book we've tried to acknowledge and address these issues. Our aim was to make the reader think even just a little about their own perceptions of ageing, their attitudes to older people, the evidence and theory base for their practice and, most importantly, to consider their practice from the perspectives of older people. We've tried to do this by providing an understanding of mental health issues in later life, a sound theoretical basis and lots of case studies and examples of evidence-based good practice. We use this approach in our own teaching and it seems to work, because it always creates a lot of discussion and debate. As our students come from a wide range of disciplines, we believe that this approach will be useful not only for those working in mental health promotion with older people, but also for those who are working in related areas such as housing or transport who would like to gain an understanding of how their work might help to promote older people's mental well-being.

Mima Cattan

## Clare in the community Harry Venning

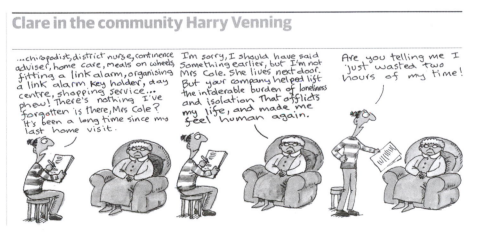

# Acknowledgements

First, my thanks go to all those older people I have worked with over the years who have given me such insights into what it's like to grow old. I would like to thank the contributors for their part in the development and completion of this text, and I am particularly indebted to Denise Forte, Liz Aitchison and Sylvia Tilford who ended up 'going that extra mile'. My thanks also go to my colleagues at Leeds Metropolitan University for their encouragement, advice and support. In particular I would like to thank Gianfranco Giuntoli, James Woodall, Rachael Dixey and Sylvia Tilford for writing their case studies about specific groups of older people. I am very grateful to Harry Venning and Guardian News and Media limited for allowing us to use 'Clare in the Community' to illustrate the plight of many older people today.

Finally, I would like to give a special thank you to Richard for making lots of cups of coffee and for helping out with the laborious proofreading at the end.

# List of abbreviations

| | |
|---|---|
| AIDS | Acquired Immunodeficiency Syndrome |
| BGOP | Better Government for Older People |
| CEC | Commission of the European Communities |
| DH | Department of Health |
| DIY | do it yourself |
| ELSA | English Longitudinal Study on Ageing |
| EMPIRIC | Ethnic Minority Psychiatric Illness Rates in the Community |
| ESAW | European Study of Ageing Well |
| ESRC | Economic and Social Research Council |
| EU | European Union |
| GNH | gross national happiness |
| GNP | gross national product |
| GP | general practitioner |
| GRR | generalized resistive resources |
| HIV | Human Immunodeficiency Virus |
| LTC | long-term condition |
| MOOTS | Moving Out Of The Shadows |
| NICE | National Institute for Health and Clinical Excellence |
| NSF | National Service Framework |
| OECD | Organisation for Economic Co-operation and Development |
| OWN | Older Women's Network |
| POPPS | Partnership for Older People's Projects |
| RCT | randomized controlled trial |
| SES | socio-economic status |
| SHAPE | Senior Health Alliance Promoting Exercise |
| SOC | sense of coherence |
| SPA | State Pension Age |
| U3A | University of the 3rd Age |
| UK | United Kingdom |
| UNESCO | United Nations Educational, Scientific and Cultural Organization |
| UNPF | United Nations Population Fund |
| US/USA | United States/of America |
| WHO | World Health Organization |

# 1 Introduction
## Mima Cattan

Ask a younger person to think about what mental health means in later life and the most likely answer is 'Dementia'. Ask an older person the same question and the response will be quite different. A survey in Scotland found that keeping active, maintaining independence and having a role in life, physical health, attitudes and values, and coping with loss were key factors in mental health (Bostock and Millar 2003). The survey suggests that for many older people mental health and well-being are not about illness, but rather something that enables them to look forward to the day and enjoy life. Before exploring these notions further we need to define 'old age'.

## What is 'old age'?

According to the World Health Organization (WHO), most countries have selected an arbitrary **chronological age** of 60 or 65 as a definition of 'older person' (WHO 2007). This age is chosen simply because it tends to be the age when most (but not all) people retire – that is retire in developed countries. We shouldn't forget that a significant proportion of older people live in developing countries, where retirement may not have the same meaning as in the UK or in other parts of the developed world. In many developing countries changes in social role and function are far more relevant 'markers' in old age than a retirement age, and such changes may come about far earlier than the notional age of 60 or 65. After all, the chronological age of 65 years was chosen by Otto von Bismark in the late nineteenth century as a retirement point, when in fact very few working adults in Germany reached the age of 65. Chronological ageing as a social construct therefore has different meanings in different countries and in different societies and cultures. We could argue that viewed as a social construct, chronological age is more attuned to a person's **functional or health age** rather than simply the number of years the person has lived.

Chronological age is particularly misleading when it comes to mental health, unless we are talking specifically about dementia. Although some mental health problems seem to increase with age, this does not mean that they are inevitable consequences of ageing. Older people have, for example, a higher risk than any other age group of completed suicide. But no one would suggest that suicide is an inevitable consequence of old age. The main factors associated with suicide in older people are thought to be certain personality traits and a history of depression, physical illness and injury (O'Connell et al. 2004; Koponen et al. 2007). The prevalence of dementia does increase with age, with figures suggesting prevalence rates ranging from under 2 per cent in people aged 65 to 69 years to almost a quarter of those aged 85 years and over. However, it has also been suggested that the occurrence of dementia varies between regions, countries, urban and rural areas, different ethnic groups, and so on (Ferri et al. 2005).

Similarly, depression in later life varies according to a range of factors, such as geographical area, gender and ethnicity. Depression has been found to be more common in southern than in northern Europe (Castro-Costa et al. 2007), among older women compared with older men; and in older people living in poverty (Beekman et al. 1999; McDougall et al. 2007). It would, therefore, seem that the notion of old age is a fusion of chronological, functional and social factors. Furthermore, the building blocks for mental health in later life, particularly older people's perceptions of mental health, include physical health, the availability of social support and social networks, security and 'happiness'.

While recognizing the complexities of defining 'old age', for this book we have chosen to define 'older people' as people aged 60 years and over because this is the definition that the WHO seems to have settled for. However, this definition is not an absolute, as demonstrated by the many examples throughout the chapters. We have acknowledged and accepted that policy, research and practice have differing defini- tions depending on the circumstances and where they are located. Importantly, figures show that the proportion of older people across the world is increasing at a faster rate than any other population group, due to both decreasing fertility rates and increasing life expectancy rates (UNPF 2005). It has been estimated that by 2025 almost a third of the population in developed countries will be aged 60 and over, while in developing countries this figure will be about 13 per cent. However, the greatest increase will occur in developing countries. In addition, the number of people aged 80 years and over is increasing at a rate twice (about 4 per cent) that of the population aged 60 and over (UN 2002). In the United Kingdom the growth rate for people aged 85 and over in 2006 was 5.9 per cent, reaching 1.2 million (National Statistics 2007).

## Mental health in later life

So why a book about mental health and well-being in later life? Obviously with more people reaching old age, we need to have an understanding of what mental health means in later life and what factors contribute to older people's mental well-being. Are older people's experiences of mental well-being the same or different from the experiences of other age groups? There has also been some concern that the issue of dementia has come to dominate the agenda of mental health and old age, forgetting that in fact the majority of older people do not suffer from dementia. The purpose of this book is therefore to focus on the promotion of mental health among older people and to provide a comprehensive text that considers the wider issues that impact on mental well-being in later life. In this we take a broad view of mental health and mental health promotion to illustrate clearly that mental health and associated factors go beyond the medical model of mental illness and the prevention of mental ill health. This does not mean that we ignore the significance of mental illness in later life. Far from it. Indeed, Chapters 4, 7 and 8 refer to mental illness and the prevention of mental ill health as part of demonstrating the links with mental well-being and the promotion of mental health. However, the intention is to draw the attention away from prevention and treatment of 'illness' and to focus on the promotion of 'health'. The WHO attempts to distinguish between health promotion and prevention and suggests that:

> Mental health promotion aims to promote positive mental health by increasing psychological well-being, competence and **resilience**, and by creating supporting living conditions and environments [while] ... Mental disorder prevention has as its target the reduction of symptoms and ultimately of mental disorders. It uses mental health promotion strategies as one of the means to achieve these goals. Mental health promotion when aiming to enhance positive mental health in the community may also have the secondary outcome of decreasing the incidence of mental disorders.
>
> (WHO 2004a: 17)

## Mental health promotion

Underpinning mental health promotion are the principles and theory of health promotion which could be said to promote holistic participatory approaches to health improvement and maintenance, irrespective of individual beliefs or culture by working at structural as well as individual levels (Secker 1998). However, the interpretation of these principles is wide and varied. As the different chapters in this book demonstrate, the promotion of mental well-being is not just implemented by a group of 'mental health promoters' but by a wide field of disciplines ranging from health to housing. Some might even argue that the maintenance of mental health and well-being has very little to do with health professionals and all the more to do with the physical and social environment. While this book does not subscribe to such a proposition, it is intended to provide the reader with a framework for mental health promotion in later life, which considers both **macro-** and **micro-level determinants** of mental health. Interestingly, although this is increasingly an accepted view of mental health determinants, very few documents to date reflect this concept when proposing action and intervention (see, for example, WHO 2004b; CEC 2005; Jané-Llopis and Anderson 2005). Although the WHO acknowledges the impact of the wider determinants of health on mental health, when it comes to defining and conceptualizing mental health, the greatest focus is on coping strategies, personality, **salutogenesis**, resilience and psychoanalytical factors (WHO 2004b). A growing interest in the environmental, cultural and **quality of life** influences on mental health in later life (WHO 2004b; Bowling and Gabriel 2007) has yet to be translated into practice on a wider scale.

## Special mental health issues for older people

While mental health and well-being are obviously important across all ages, some of the issues and how these are addressed in practice are unique and of greater relevance in later life, which is reflected in a large number of national and international strategy and policy documents (see, for example, DH 1999; DH 2001; Berkels et al. 2004; WHO 2004a, 2004b, 2005; Lee 2006). For example, retirement can have a major impact on the mental health of people aged 60 to 80 years. For some it can mean a time of freedom from the grind of employment, the child-rearing years and other responsibilities. It can offer an opportunity to 'do the things they hadn't had time to do before' and a chance to develop new social contacts. In some cultures reaching old age might mean increased social status. However, for others it may lead to loss of status, a perceived reduced role in life and less contact with friends and colleagues from work. Other factors that may impact on the mental health of this age group include a gradual deterioration in health and physical capability, loss of financial stability, changing environments (moving home) and a loss of the sense of 'belonging' and other social and psychological factors.

People aged 80 years and over increasingly face the loss of close friends, family and partners, deteriorating functional ability and the sense of their own purpose in life. For this reason the mental health impact may be more chronic than in 'early' old age. The fear of losing independence is common in this age group. Caring for a partner who is becoming increasingly frail or has dementia can contribute to individuals' social isolation and feelings of loneliness and abandonment. And finally, people in this age group are increasingly dealing with bereavement, dying and death, and facing their own end of life. These are of course generalizations: older people are not a homogeneous group. They vary, just as any age group, in culture, values, personal make-up, life experiences, economic status, health, and so on. And all these factors impact on their mental health and well-being. Resilience as a theoretical framework is often mentioned in these circumstances because it focuses on individual traits and supportive environments. But older people's mental wellness is more than the sum of what and who they are and how they relate to their social environment. In the survey of older people's views on what affects mental well-being in later life mentioned earlier, financial security featured strongly among the important factors (Bostock and Millar 2003). Financial security is dependent on income, pension and housing among other things and these are driven by national and international policy. Such macro-level impact on mental health goes beyond the notion of resilience.

Another issue we shouldn't forget in relation to mental health and the heterogeneity of older people is the diversity of old age. Are there special mental health and health promotion issues that we need to consider in relation to black and minority ethnic older people, older lesbians, gay men, and bisexual men and women, older prisoners, homeless people, grandparents or caregivers? The little research that is available suggests there may be. However, we should not make too many assumptions about their 'special' status because it may be that it is because they are 'invisible' that their specific mental health needs are not addressed rather than because they are *older*. The important issue here is that for mental health promotion to be responsive to the needs of these groups, it must take into account the multitude of factors that impact on their mental well-being. Being older carries some risk factors in relation to mental health: being older and homeless brings additional dimensions to this vulnerability.

## The social determinants of mental health

This book takes a holistic approach to mental health and mental health promotion based on the wider social determinants of health. It recognizes that the promotion of mental health with older people goes beyond focusing on the individual and individual risk factors at a micro level and incorporates wider macro-level environmental and ecological factors. However, simultaneously the authors acknowledge that the distinction between macro- and micro-level mental health interventions is frequently blurred. The WHO makes the point that public health policies should encompass multiple-level prevention interventions in order to address multiple causal trajectories for populations at risk (WHO 2004a). And although many will agree that we need to take into account the wider determinants of mental health and that we could question what is meant by the notion of 'populations at risk', in reality a large proportion of those working to promote the mental health and well-being of older people either focus on prevention or work in settings where the aim is to promote mental wellness of local communities and individuals within these communities. It is possible that theoretically at this level, **social capital** and ecological models may provide a framework for taking mental health promotion forward. These points are explored in this book, either through evidence and examples or through debate and discussion. Importantly, the chapters are driven by older people's perceptions and views about what matters for them in mental health and how best to promote mental well-being and mental wellness in later life (Bostock and Millar 2003; Age Concern and Mental Health Foundation 2006).

## The structure of the book

The first three chapters provide a framework for the ensuing chapters. They do this by describing and discussing current issues around definitions of age and ageing and the theories – social gerontology and health promotion – that help us to understand mental health and mental health promotion in later life and the way policy and practice shape our understanding of mental health promotion in later life. Chapter 2 in particular explores and discusses the debates around what is meant by mental health and well-being, and mental illness and the determinants of mental health. It also considers older people's own perspectives on mental well-being and importantly any distinctive mental health issues that may arise for the hidden groups of older people, such as older people in prison, carers or refugees and asylum seekers. Such issues are important when considering the direction of mental health promoting interventions and the evidence base because this recognizes the diversity among older people. Chapter 3 reviews and discusses theory as part of **evidence-based practice** in mental health promotion. It not only considers theory as constructed through academic concepts but also in what way theory-driven mental health promotion relates to lay perspectives of mental health and well-being. Chapter 4 moves away from concepts and theory, and focuses on the debates around public versus individual approaches and lay versus professional perspectives. In addition, it explores the evidence base for promoting mental health compared with preventing mental ill health in later life.

Chapters 5 to 8 have 'loosely' been called older people's perspectives of mental health. This is because the four chapters were derived from older people's views and thoughts on mental health (Bostock and Millar 2003; Age Concern and Mental Health Foundation 2006). These themes are the impact of retirement in terms of financial security, the role of maintaining physical and mental activity, sensory impairment and the wider environment, and independence and control. Each chapter provides the policy context for the theme and addresses the associations with mental health in later life in different cultural settings. In addition a strong emphasis is on the evidence base for effective interventions to promote mental health, with a range of theory-driven evidence-based examples from the UK as well as from other countries. The purpose of these chapters is to give the reader a strong sense of what the main mental health issues are for older people in a variety of settings, cultures and population groups, and to provide accessible, evidence-led examples of good mental health promotion practice. Finally, the concluding chapter will explore the future of promoting mental health in later life in relation to political will and resource implications by drawing together and reflecting on the main themes and messages in the book.

With such breadth of subject matter to cover, the contributors come from a diverse backgrounds. In fact one might say that some of the contributors are not from what one would think of as 'traditional' mental health promoting backgrounds, academically or professionally. This of course demonstrates how mental health promotion in relation to older people is arguably everybody's business. More importantly for the reader, however, the authors bring their perspectives on the factors that impact on mental well-being in later life and draw on their experiences and rich knowledge base to put forward sound proposals for the promotion of mental wellness among older people. This diversity should also provide a platform for some interesting and creative debates about where the priorities should be with regards to maintaining a mentally well population of older people.

## In conclusion

In an interview shortly before her death in 2004, Margaret Simey, aged 97, reflected on the 'appalling feeling of isolation and the terrible sense of insecurity', and 'the crushing boredom of life, busy though it keeps me' (Owen 2005: 28), following a deterioration in her physical health, combined with services that didn't fit and an environment that she was no longer able to be part of. She had been a life-long campaigner for social justice and an activist for the rights of older people. Reading her story it would be easy to assume that her feelings of frustration and insecurity were simply as a result of her loss of mobility. However, Margaret Simey was an astute woman and what she really described was an environment that had become alien to her, an environment that no longer had space for older people. And that, combined with her own frailty, contributed to her feelings of isolation and boredom. Perhaps the most important way to promote the mental health and well-being of older people is to transform our social, cultural and external environment to one that is inclusive and provides space for older people.

# References

Age Concern and Mental Health Foundation (2006) *Promoting Mental Health and Well-being in Later Life: A First Report from the UK Inquiry into Mental Health and Well-Being in Later Life*. London: Age Concern and Mental Health Foundation.

Beekman, A. T., Copeland, J. R. and Prince, M. J. (1999) Review of community prevalence of depression in later life, *The British Journal of Psychiatry*, 174: 307–11.

Berkels, H., Henderson, J., Henke, N. et al. (2004) *Mental Health Promotion and Prevention Strategies for Coping with Anxiety, Depression and Stress Related Disorders in Europe Final Report 2001–2003*. Dortmund/Berlin/Dresden: Federal Institute for Occupational Safety and Health.

Bostock, Y. and Millar, C. (2003) *Older People's Perceptions of the Factors that Affect Mental Well-Being in Later Life*. Edinburgh: NHS Health Scotland.

Bowling, A. and Gabriel, Z. (2007) Lay theories of quality of life in older age, *Ageing and Society*, 27(6): 827–48.

Castro-Costa, E., Dewey, M., Stewart, R. et al. (2007) Prevalence of depressive symptoms and syndromes in later life in ten European countries, *The British Journal of Psychiatry*, 191: 393–401.

CEC (Commission of the European Communities) (2005) *Improving the Mental Health of the Population: Towards a Strategy on Mental Health for the European Union*. Brussels: European Union.

DH (Department of Health) (1999) *Mental Health National Service Framework*. London: HMSO.

DH (Department of Health) (2001) *National Service Framework for Older People*. London: HMSO.

Ferri, C. P., Prince, M., Brayne, C. et al. (2005) Global prevalence of dementia: a Delphi consensus study, *The Lancet*, 366: 2112–17.

Jané-Llopis, E. and Anderson, P. (2005) *Mental Health Promotion and Mental Disorder Prevention: A Policy for Europe*. Nijmegen: Radboud University, Nijmegen.

Koponen, H. J., Viilo, K., Hakko, H. et al. (2007) Rates and previous disease history in old age suicide, *International Journal of Geriatric Psychiatry*, Doi:10.1002/gps.1651.

Lee, M. (2006) *Promoting Mental Health and Well-Being in Later Life*. London: Age Concern and Mental Health Foundation.

McDougall, F. A., Kvaal, K., Mathews, F. E. et al. (2007) Prevalence of depression in older people in England and Wales: the MRC CFA study, *Psychological Medicine*, Doi:10.1017/S0033291707000372.

National Statistics (2007) *Ageing*. Available at: http://www.statistics.gov.uk/cci/nugget.asp?ID=949 (accessed 5 Jan. 2008).

O'Connell, H., Chin, A. V., Cunningham, C., and Lawlor, B. A. (2004) Recent developments: suicide in older people, *British Medical Journal*, 329: 895–9.

Owen, T. (2005) *Dying in Older Age*. London: Help the Aged.

Secker, J. (1998) Current conceptualizations of mental health and mental health promotion, *Health Education Research*, 13(1): 57–66.

UN (United Nations) (2002) *World Population Ageing: 1950–2050*. New York: Population Division, Department of Economic and Social Affairs.

UNPF (United Nations Population Fund) (2005) *Population Ageing – A Larger and Older Population*. New York: UNPF. Available at: http://www.unfpa.org/pds/ageing.htm. (accessed 5 Jan. 2008).

WHO (World Health Organisation) (2004a) *Prevention of Mental Disorders: Effective Interventions and Policy Options*. Geneva: WHO.

WHO (World Health Organisation) (2004b) *Promoting Mental Health: Concepts – Emerging Evidence*. Geneva: WHO.

WHO (World Health Organisation) (2005) *Mental Health Action Plan for Europe: Facing the Challenges, Building Solutions*, European Ministerial Conference on Mental Health, Helsinki.

WHO (World Health Organization) (2007) *Definition of an Older or Elderly Person*. Available at: http://www.who.int/healthinfo/survey/ageingdefnolder/en/ index.html, (accessed 7 Nov. 2007).

# 2 What is mental health and mental well-being?
## Gill Windle

## Editor's foreword

Before going on to consider areas of mental health promotion in later life we need to agree what we mean by mental health and mental well-being. Building on a **systematic review** this chapter starts by discussing definitions of mental health and well-being. It goes on to explore in what way quality of life issues are related to mental well-being and how culture impacts on the way we view mental health in later life. A major and important section of the chapter defines and reviews age-associated determinants of well-being, demonstrating clearly the breadth of factors that impact on mental well-being in old age. Linked to this the author discusses the 'well-being paradox', which suggests that there is a positive relationship between increasing age and subjective well-being despite increasing risk of poor health. The chapter concludes with a useful overview of some of the theories that have been developed to explain mental well-being.

## Introduction

Despite the common use of the terms 'mental health' or 'mental well-being' in research, policy, practice and everyday life, defining what exactly we mean by these terms appears to be somewhat of a challenge. Taking up this theme, this chapter presents some definitions and key conceptualizations of mental health and mental well-being, emphasizing the focus on positive psychological functioning. Following that, some of the main determinants of mental well-being are discussed. The resilience of older age is then examined from a psychological perspective, focusing on how mental well-being might be maintained when other conditions in life are less than desirable.

## Definitions and conceptualizations of mental health and well-being

Research with groups of people aged 50–90 in Britain found that when asked to define mental well-being in a simple statement, most found it very difficult (Bostock and

Millar 2003). One of the groups suggested that mental well-being related to the importance of having goals and aims in life: 'having something to get up for in the morning' (2003: 7.1). However, other research with people aged 50+ reports that when asked to define mental health and well-being, the majority (42 per cent) described it from the perspective of mental illness, referring to dementia or Alzheimer's disease. Fewer respondents saw the terms from a positive perspective with 19 per cent citing 'healthy mind', 15 per cent citing healthy body, 12 per cent referring to happiness and 10 per cent defining it as being able to cope with life and being in control (Francis and Allgar 2005: 14). In these instances it is apparent that the participants view mental health and mental well-being as either negative or positive psychological functioning. Importantly, the notion and meaning of mental health vary across cultures (see Box 2.1), with many of whose languages simply not having an expression for 'mental health'.

---

**Box 2.1** Examples of the meaning of mental health in different cultures

In South Africa, a public survey showed that most people thought mental illnesses were related to either stress or a lack of willpower rather than to medical disorders. Contrary to expectations, levels of stigma were higher in urban areas and among people with higher levels of education (WHO 2007).

A study among urban Xhosa-speaking South African found that they had limited understanding of bio-medically constructed dementia. The terms used to describe dementia pertained to four main areas: bewitchment, where mental illness is seen as being possessed by evil spirits; madness; behaviour; and some expressions borrowed from Western medicine (Ferreira and Makoni 2002).

In some South Asian cultures mental illness is thought to come from somebody having looked at you with the 'evil eye' or jealously.

In many cultures mental health and mental illness are tied to your destiny, which means that you can do very little to change it. In Buddhist and Hindu religion, mental illness can be attributed to the belief in Karma, which means that your illness is due to something you have done in your past causing conflict and problems (O'Mahony and Connelly 2007).

In rural Thailand animist concepts co-exist with Buddhism. According to animist beliefs, mental illness is caused by bad spirits and because Kwan, the 'life spirit', has left the body. However, through meditation Buddhists believe that Kwan can return (Burnard et al. 2007).

---

This lack of clarity around what exactly mental health is has also been reflected in mental health research. Ryff and Singer (1996) describe how the meaning of concepts such as mental health are generally negatively biased, with a focus on the absence of disease rather than the presence of positive conditions. The investigation of positive psychological functioning has also received less attention. A review of the literature found that research publications address negative, rather than positive psychological states in a ratio of 17 to one (Diener et al. 1999). The 2006 UK Inquiry into Mental Health and Well-Being in Later Life (Lee 2006) also suggests that the promotion of mental well-being has traditionally been neglected in favour of promoting physical health. Yet there is a strong interplay between the two which is recognized in the World Health Organization's (WHO) definition, where health is defined as 'a complete state of physical, mental and social well-being and not merely the absence of disease or infirmity' (2007: 3). Philosophical writings show that the search for a life of well-being – 'the good life' – is ancient, yet it is only relatively recently that it has been systematically measured and studied (Diener et al. 1997). Therefore attempts to investigate well-being scientifically are relatively new.

An early position on positive mental health was developed by Jahoda (1958) who suggested six criteria:

1 Sense of identity, including self-acceptance, self-esteem and self-reliance.
2 Investment in living and in realizing one's potential.
3 Unifying outlook and sense of meaning and purpose in life.
4 Autonomy, including self-determination with respect to demands from society.
5 Accurate perception of reality and sensitivity to others.
6 Mastery of the environment, manifested in interpersonal relationships, engagement in work and play, and ability to solve problems.

A number of these criteria are reflected in more recent descriptions of mental health. Although there are no consistently used definitions, the World Health Organization (2005: 2) describes mental health as: 'a state of well-being in which every individual realises his or her own potential, can cope with the normal stresses of life, can work productively and fruitfully, and is able to make a contribution to her or his community'. An earlier definition in the 1986 Ottawa Charter for health promotion states that: 'mental health is the emotional and spiritual resilience which allows us to enjoy life and to survive pain, disappointment and sadness. It is a positive sense of well-being and an underlying belief in our own, and others' dignity and worth' (WHO 1986).

These definitions suggest that the definition of a mentally healthy state is far broader than simply that of not having a mental illness or disorder; they do not explicitly refer to mental disorders such as clinical depression. In these descriptions mental health is attained through the presence of attributes that promote positive psychological functioning. Such definitions indicate that mental health reflects a life with quality. They also highlight the importance of resilience and coping, remaining active and involved, and social capital. Drawing on these definitions, the following section briefly outlines a number of factors that have been conceptualized as being important to mental health.

## Positive aspects of mental health

Quality of life is an important concept to consider in understanding mental health. Like mental health there is no accepted consistent definition of quality of life, and the term is often used interchangeably with that of well-being (Haug and Folmar 1986; Smith 2000). It is generally regarded as a multidimensional construct encompassing a wide range of factors such as health, housing, income, social networks along with subjective perceptions of these factors and perceptions of well-being. As an example of this, a survey of 999 people aged 65 and over living in their own homes in Britain identified seven key determinants of a good quality of life (Bowling et al. 2003). These were:

- Having good social relationships with family, friends and neighbours;
- Having social roles and participating in social and voluntary activities, plus other activities/hobbies performed alone;
- Having good health and functional ability;
- Living in a good home and neighbourhood;
- Having a positive outlook and psychological well-being;
- Having adequate income;
- Maintaining independence and control over one's life.

However, the subjective assessment of well-being is often used in research to indicate quality of life and this places it within the framework of positive mental functioning.

Another commonly referred to component is subjective well-being. Subjective well-being refers to the individual experience of evaluating life in positive terms (Diener 1984). For example Diener et al. (1999) define subjective well-being as 'a broad category of phenomena that includes people's emotional responses, domain satisfactions and global judgements about life satisfaction' (1999: 227). Subjective well-being is considered an important component of 'the good life' (Lawton 1983; Ryff and Keyes 1995; Diener et al. 1999; Smith 2000), with positive outcomes considered to be an indicator of successful ageing (Bowling 1991).

Positive affect and negative affect represent the emotional/mood component of subjective well-being. Positive affect can be divided into specific mood states such as happiness, affection, interested, etc. Negative affect reflects mood states such as shame, guilt and sadness. The subjective assessment of satisfaction with one's life focuses on what enables people to evaluate their lives in terms of positive experiences – a cognitive judgement (Diener 1984; Diener et al. 1997). Life satisfaction has been the focus of much research in gerontology, representing an indicator of quality of life and successful ageing. It is this subjective assessment of well-being which is argued by Bond and Corner (2004) to represent the most important domain of quality of life.

Personality traits and resources – that is the characteristics or qualities within the individual which predispose the person to behave in characteristic ways across a range of situations – are also implicated in good mental health and well-being. Such resources can promote a sense of control, coping and adaptation in older age (Baltes and Baltes 1986; Lachman 1986; Ryff and Singer 1996). It is suggested that these personal qualities have a developmental trajectory, being acquired over the lifespan (Ryff and Singer 1996). Personality resources are suggested to protect individuals in the face of adversity and lead to positive adaptive behaviour by acting as a 'buffer' (Rutter 1987) or as compensatory factors which directly influence outcomes (Masten 1999).

## Culture, mental health and well-being

It is important to recognize that these concepts of mental health primarily reflect theoretical developments in Western cultures where mental ill health is now becoming more widely recognized. In contrast to this it is suggested that there is low awareness regarding mental illness and the importance of mental health in many communities in developing countries. Ageing in developing nations can be a considerable challenge where there are falling levels of family support and little if any social welfare.

It would appear that limited research has been undertaken in developing nations around the meaning of mental health and well-being. In addition, there are methodological considerations when investigating mental health in such countries. We cannot assume that our Western conceptualizations will be the same as those in other parts of the world. Western concepts of mental health and well-being are very much dependent on individual, personal qualities. In contrast, in other countries such as China, mental health and well-being are more likely to reflect a **collectivist** perspective, reflecting religious beliefs stemming from, for example, Buddhism and Taoism (Box 2.2.).

---

**Box 2.2** Happiness in the Himalayas

Bhutan is the only country in the world that measures its success by gross national happiness (GNH) as opposed to gross national product (GNP). Inner spiritual development is considered as equally important as material development, reflecting the country's Buddhist philosophy. Material and technological advances are not rejected but they must be balanced against human values. Television was only introduced in 1999 – and wrestling was not broadcasted as it was felt to offer little to promote happiness! Care of the environment is paramount. Individuals with a grievance can obtain a direct appointment with the King himself. Happiness surveys indicate the people of Bhutan are some of the happiest in the world, with it being ranked eighth out of 178 countries (White 2007).

---

## Age-associated determinants of well-being

A key question in any research on mental health in older age is how people maintain well-being if other conditions in their lives are less than desirable. In older age there is an increased potential for negative experiences which could threaten well-being; ageing can be associated with losses and changes in a number of life domains (Baltes and Mayer 1999).

---

**Box 2.3** Key facts about older age

- The prevalence of late onset dementia increases with age, doubling every five years from 1.3 per cent for 65–69 years to 32.5 per cent for 95+ years.
- Limiting long-standing illness increases with age, from 20 per cent of men and women aged 50–54 to over 70 per cent of those aged 85 and over.
- Mobility problems were reported by 68 per cent of women and 52 per cent of men aged 85 and over living in private households.
- In the General Household Survey, 31 per cent of the total number of carers are aged 60 or over.
- In older age there is an increased likelihood of the bereavement of a spouse or close friends, which in turn can result in social isolation and loneliness (Wenger et al. 1996).
- Older people in receipt of a pension are more likely to experience continual low income than their younger counterparts. In Scotland, 32 per cent of people who had reached state pension age did not feel they had enough money to live on.
- Women outnumber men by four to three at the age of 65 or over and by almost two to one at the age of 80 or over (UN, 2001).
- Older women are also more likely to be widowed, live alone, have a lower average gross income than older men and be more dependent upon benefits.
- Isolation and loneliness – one in five people over 65 are alone for more than 12 hours a day.

---

There is a substantial amount of research that has examined the inter-relationships between aspects of later life and mental health concepts. This section focuses on some of the key determinants highlighted in other recent robust pieces of research.

### Quality of life

A review of the international quality of life literature by Bowling (2004) was undertaken to classify the wide-ranging approaches taken towards examining the concept. It focused on the literature driven by theory or other research (as opposed to literature derived from the voices of older people themselves). It reported that the most frequently reported associations with well-being or quality of life in older age are good health and functional ability, a feeling of usefulness or adequacy; social participation; friends and social support, and a good level of income or other indicator of socio-economic status (Bowling 2004: 8).

An accompanying systematic review focusing on the factors nominated by older people themselves was undertaken so as to draw comparisons with those identified in the previous literature review (Brown and Flynn 2004). The review found that the main factors regarded as important for quality of life were family relationships, relationships with others, happiness, religion/spirituality, independence/mobility/autonomy, health, social/leisure activities and finance/standard of living (Brown and Flynn 2004).

Drawing on policy and literature reviews, together with the views of almost 900 older people and carers, organizations and professionals, the UK Inquiry into Mental Health and Well-Being (Lee 2006) highlights five main areas that affect mental health and well-being in later life – discrimination, participation in meaningful activity, relationships, physical health and poverty.

These reviews indicate a general consensus of some of the key factors associated with subjective well-being reflecting those nominated by older people themselves and those derived from theory and research. They also highlight the importance of a number of areas (such as social relationships and networks, participation, etc.) that contribute to the concept of 'social capital' discussed in other chapters. However, an important distinction between the two is the inclusion of religion/spirituality in the review by Brown and Flynn (2004). In addition, neither review reports or discusses research that has examined the impact of cognitive impairment or dementia.

## Cognitive impairment

The evidence for the relationship between cognitive impairment and life satisfaction indicates that more research has focused on negative psychological symptoms (depression) than positive psychological outcomes. Depressive symptoms have been associated with cognitive decline (Teri and Wagner 1992) and it is reported that depression is common in people with dementia: prevalence rates have been estimated at approximately 30 per cent (Ballard et al. 1995). More recently a study of people aged 65 and over with dementia found that 40.2 per cent of the respondents were depressed according to the Cornell scale for depression in dementia (Waite et al. 2004). Using a subjective assessment of quality of life – the Dementia Quality of Life Scale and the Geriatric Depression Scale – it is reported that dementia patients with greater depressive symptoms rated their quality of life as low (Sands et al. 2004).

In contrast, an Australian survey of community dwelling people aged 75 and over found that cognitive impairment did not predict life satisfaction or depression (Broe et al. 1998). However, this study differed from the others in that it specifically excluded people with a diagnosis of dementia. Further evidence for the relationship between cognitive impairment and life satisfaction was found in a German study. Respondents with mild cognitive impairment reported lower life satisfaction that those with normal cognitive function (Morawetz et al. 2001), however, in this study the sample size was low (26 in each group) limiting any generalizations.

One of the main difficulties associated with evaluating the well-being of someone with cognitive impairment is that the nature of their disorder can affect the accuracy of their own rating. Likewise inaccuracies from caregivers' assessments can also present discrepancies. Consequently self-ratings may underestimate the extent of depression in comparison with carers or clinicians (Teri and Wagner 1992). Despite methodological difficulties, cognitive impairment is a correlate of older age that needs to be considered in its relationship to subjective well-being.

## Gender

Gender is another potential risk factor that was not identified in the reviews. In 14 European countries, being widowed or separated was associated with an increase in depressive symptoms (Prince et al. 1999). In reviewing the literature Diener et al. (1999) report that while female gender is consistently associated with depression, the same is not always found for subjective well-being, and men and women appear to be approximately equal. More recent findings support this trend. No significant differences in life satisfaction were found between males and females or for age groups (aged 70 +) (Windle and Woods 2004). In contrast, a **meta-analysis** of 300 studies reports that women had slightly lower life satisfaction than men, although the effects were small explaining less than 1 per cent of the variance in well-being (Pinquart and Sörensen 2001). However, these authors had a lower age limit for inclusion (55+). Also a quarter of the studies they identified could not be included as they did not report correlations. Further analysis suggested that it was the gender differences in physical health, marital status and socio-economic status (SES) that were likely to have consequences for psychological functioning, and not gender *per se* (Pinquart and Sörensen 2001).

## Ethnicity

There are some clear associations between ethnicity and mental health. A particularly useful large-scale source of data in the UK is the *Ethnic Minority Psychiatric Illness Rates in the Community* (EMPIRIC) survey (Sproston and Nazroo 2002), which consists of two elements: a quantitative survey of rates of mental illness among Black Caribbean, Indian, Pakistani, Bangladeshi, Chinese and Irish people in England and a qualitative study of the same groups investigating ethnic and cultural differences in the context, experience and expression of mental distress. The study found that common mental disorders increased with age among Pakistani and Bangladeshi men and Indian women, while across all ages rates were significantly higher among Pakistani and Bangladeshi women. Cultural differences between ethnic groups in presentation of symptoms of mental ill health have been reported, for example, the greater tendency of South Asian women to present with physical rather than mental symptoms which may not be picked up by doctors or other health workers (Nazroo 1997). This may in part be due to a reluctance in South Asian communities to report mental health problems due to the stigmatization of such conditions (Gupta 1992; Nazroo 1997). There are also problems because of cultural bias in diagnosis of mental health problems (Knowles 1991; McCracken et al. 1997). A study from the USA reports that black Americans had less psychological distress in comparison to their white counterparts (Kahana et al. 1995).

# The well-being paradox

The previous section has highlighted areas of life where being part of a disadvantaged population, losses and changes can have an adverse effect on well-being. However, there is evidence that subjective well-being can remain relatively stable over time. A survey of almost 60,000 adults in 40 nations found that life satisfaction actually increased slightly from the 20s into the 80s, with little variation in the eldest two decades (Diener and Suh 1997). Other research has found that the subjective well-being scores of older adults are often in the same range as those of younger people (Baltes 1993). This disparity in the positive relationship between increasing age and subjective well-being, despite the increasing influence of risk factors such as poor health, has been termed the 'well-being paradox' (Staudinger 2000) or the 'satisfaction paradox' (Diener et al. 1999). As an example, the following section focuses on the role of physical health. It summarizes some of the contradictory evidence for the impact of health on well-being. Drawing on theory and research it presents a model for maintaining mental well-being.

A recent survey in Scotland found that good health was cited as most important in having a happy older age in both younger and older respondents (Scottish Executive 2006). Reductions in physical health, physical functioning and most health problems have been linked to poor and worsening levels of life satisfaction (Bowling et al. 1993; Bowling et al. 1997). Yet the potential negative experiences of ageing such as failing health are not consistently associated with reduced subjective well-being. A **longitudinal study** by Brief et al. (1993) failed to find a direct effect of objective health (doctor visits and hospitalization) on life satisfaction, but it was predicted by a subjective assessment of health. It is an often found paradox that older people regularly report their health as good in spite of some impairment (Siddell 1995). This is supported in recent evidence from Wales. In a study of 421 people aged 70 and over, although 61 per cent reported a limiting long-standing illness or disability, 8 per cent reported their health as excellent, 31 per cent as very good, 33 per cent as good, 24 per cent as fair and only 4 per cent as poor (Burholt et al. 2003). This suggests that the impact of disability on well-being may depend more on the perception of the situation.

There are theoretical perspectives that help explain the well-being paradox and that highlight the role of regulatory mechanisms that are central to the individual. Top–down theory (Diener 1984) predicts that aspects central to the individual's personality influence the way a person might react to situations and life changes such as ill health. It is likely that ongoing efforts to cope with, and adapt to, factors such as ill health or a reduction in activities will occur in order to maintain acceptable levels of well-being. Consequently a positive interpretation facilitated through the individual's personality could maintain acceptable levels of well-being, although this might not necessarily reflect their actual situation. To illustrate this point, the following presents some primary data (Windle 2006).

The data were collected in a **cross-sectional survey** as part of the European Study of Ageing Well (ESAW) in 2003. Six West European countries participated in the study: Austria, Italy, Luxembourg, the Netherlands, Sweden and Britain. The following analyses reflect the British data, which were drawn from 1847 people in England,

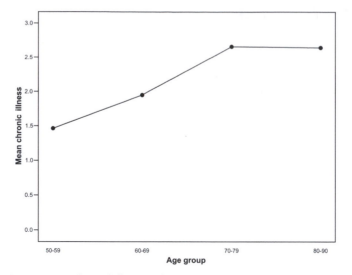

**Figure 2.1**  Average number of illnesses by age group
*Source*: ESAW data

Wales and Scotland aged 50–90. The full ESAW questionnaire covered a wide range of areas – social support, health, activities, psychological factors and material resources. Twenty-six items assessed the presence of chronic disorders. The analysis show that as age increased there was also a significant increase in their number of chronic illnesses ($F(3,1839) = 41.30$, $P < 0.001$; see Figure 2.1).

However, in response to a question 'How do you rate your own health?', there were no significant differences for the categories of self-reported health between and within each of the age groups. Across the whole sample less than 10 per cent reported their health as poor (see Figure 2.2). The highest proportions reporting their health as poor or fair were the 70–79 age group. In comparison to the other age groups the 80–90 year olds had the highest proportion reporting their health as good, despite a higher average number of chronic illnesses.

Figure 2.3 shows that although the most favourable ratings of own health were given by respondents with low levels of chronic illness, over one-third (37 per cent) of those with higher than average number of chronic illnesses reported their health as either good or excellent. These findings imply that the individuals' perception was portrayed far more positively than that of their actual health status. The following presents a theoretical perspective to further explain this disparity.

## Psychological factors as a mechanism to maintaining mental well-being

Earlier in this chapter personality traits/psychological resources were highlighted as being important for good mental health and well-being. Here this position is expanded. A short selection of literature is presented and a hypothesis tested using the ESAW data.

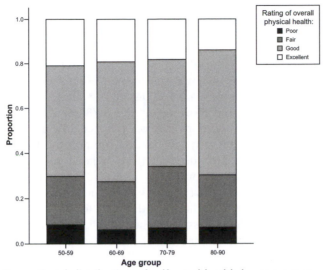

**Figure 2.2** Proportional distribution of self-rated health by age group
*Source*: ESAW data

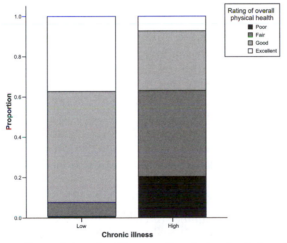

**Figure 2.3** Perceptions of own health according to levels of chronic illness
*Source*: SAW data

In terms of the Stress Process Model (Pearlin et al. 1981), personality resources could protect individuals in the face of adversity and lead to positive adaptive behaviour by moderating or 'buffering' the effects of stressors such as failing health. In the context of the model of selective optimization with compensation, how individuals can deal with ageing and the age-related tendency for increased losses and fewer gains are determined by regulatory processes (Baltes 1993). Consequently the moderating influence of the self/personality may compensate for change or adversity.

Continuity theory also emphasizes the importance of inner resources such as the personality/self, goals and coping strategies to maintain satisfaction with life despite changes in health, functioning and social circumstances (Atchley 1989).

Research that has examined the influence that psychological resources have on well-being finds that they can have an intervening effect. They can increase the possibility of positive changes in health behaviours and well-being (Wells and Kendig 1999), or they can limit the potential negative influences on well-being of risk factors associated with ageing (Windle and Woods 2004). In the latter study, a representative sample of 420 people aged 70 and above (mean age = 78) were interviewed in North Wales. The impact of a number of factors on the person's life satisfaction were examined, and it emerged that physical health limitations, loneliness, housing difficulties and being widowed or divorced were related to lower levels of life satisfaction. However, when the person's sense of environmental mastery (measured on a nine-item scale developed by Ryff 1989) was included in the predictive model, this mitigated the effects of both physical health limitations and housing difficulties, and, to a lesser extent, of loneliness. In other words, having a strong sense of environmental mastery reduced the impact of the difficult circumstances the older person was experiencing.

The impact of other psychological resources on well-being has also been evaluated. In a systematic review of the literature a person's sense of coherence was found to be strongly associated with a range of other psychological resources and indicators of mental health (Eriksson and Lindström 2005). According to the salutogenic theory of health, there are a range of factors that seem to play a role in helping the people cope and survive. Antonovsky (1987) called these generalized resistive resources (GRRs). These are the properties of a person (or a collective) which have facilitated successful coping with the inherent stressors of human existence. The GRRs foster repeated life experiences that help someone to see the world as *making sense* cognitively, instrumentally or emotionally, contributing to or creating a sense of coherence (SOC). Antonovsky defined SOC as 'a global orientation that expresses the extent to which one has a pervasive, enduring though dynamic, feeling of confidence that one's internal and external environments are predictable and that there is a high probability that things will work out as well as can reasonably be expected' (1987: xiii.).

Mastery has been found to improve mental health and functioning (Badger 1993, 2001). Increases in mental health and life satisfaction scores were found to be associated with respondents who had higher internal locus of control (Landau and Litwin 2001). Control beliefs have been associated with well-being between the ages of 25 and 75 (Lachman and Weaver 1998). Other research has found that older adults demonstrate no reduction in psychological resources central to the self such as self-esteem or sense of personal control despite losses in functioning and the perception of such losses (Baltes and Baltes 1986; Lachman 1986). The beneficial effect of self-efficacy is demonstrated in research which shows self-efficacy to diminish the negative impact of impaired functional capacity on depressive symptoms (Knipscheer et al. 2000). Self-efficacy has also been found to buffer the impact of cancer on depressive symptoms in people aged between 55 and 85 (Bisschop et al. 2004). The beneficial effects of such resources in older age may then be a key factor for well-being.

## Psychological resilience

Other research that has examined resources such as mastery, self-esteem and optimism has conceptualized them as part of the core of the reserve capacity that provides a basis of resilience in older age (Gallo et al. 2005). Psychological resilience is thought to be important in later life as a component of successful psychosocial adjustment (Wagnild and Young 1993). In that respect, resilience is important for positive mental health in older age. Conceptually, it was derived from observations that although exposed to substantial stressors and risks, people can still function positively and recover quickly from set-backs (Rutter 1995). In recent work, Windle et al. (2008) examined a theoretical and empirical model of psychological resilience, where resilience is comprised of self-esteem, competence and control. Using this measure of resilience, the following analysis examines how it may intervene in the potentially negative relationship between ill health and well-being.

The analyses examine this position using the moderating hypothesis (see Figure 2.4). This hypothesis states that a moderator variable is one that influences the direction and/or strength of the relation between an independent variable and a dependent variable (Baron and Kenny 1986). In this context it is hypothesized that the presence of resilience in the face of the chronic illness stressor will provide a compensatory mechanism that results in the optimization of subjective well-being. For these analyses the Life Satisfaction Index (Wood et al. 1969) represents the outcome of subjective well-being. The scale was developed for use with older populations and different ethnic groups, and is commonly used to measure well-being in gerontology research. It is a 13-item global measure of past, present and future states and is considered to be an indication of successful aging. Respondents were asked whether they agreed or disagreed with each of the items relating to satisfaction with life. Each item is scored 0, 1 or 2, with the total score ranging from 0–26.

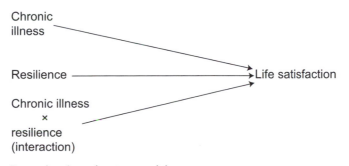

**Figure 2.4** Example of moderator model

Multiple regression procedures were used to assess moderation. In the following analyses the moderation hypotheses are supported if the interaction (between illness and resilience) is significant while controlling for the main effects of the predictor and the moderator. Age, gender and education levels are also included as control variables.

Prior to including the interaction term there was a significant main effect of chronic illness on life satisfaction for all of the age groups (results not shown). A moderating effect of resilience on the chronic illness–well-being link was found in all of the age groups except the 50–59-year-olds (see Figure 2.5). For those with increasing numbers of chronic illnesses an associated increase in life satisfaction was found when resilience was higher. But, for all, higher levels of life satisfaction were related to higher levels of resilience and lower levels of illness. The lowest levels of life satisfaction were associated with a combination of lower levels of resilience and higher levels of illness.

## Conclusions

This chapter aimed to provide some indication as to what exactly is meant by mental health and well-being from both a theoretical perspective and that of older people themselves. It is clear that mental health is more than the absence of illness. To be mentally healthy requires positive psychological functioning, which is a product of a person's satisfaction with life and happiness, and their personality resources such as self-esteem, competence, control and resilience. In turn, variations in positive psychological functioning are strongly influenced by the multiple factors that contribute to overall quality of life in older age. These include health, functional ability, social resources, material resources, participation in meaningful activities, religion/spirituality and cognitive functioning. Older people have stated that lack of participation in society leads to marginalization, low esteem and low status (Higgs 1995). Consequently, an improvement in well-being may be implied if older people were given the appropriate opportunities for participation.

Discrimination in terms of ethnicity and gender is often a disadvantage for good mental health. Discrimination is highlighted in the UK Inquiry as being a key determinant of poor mental health, with age discrimination being a common experience in later life. Racism is also an important factor. It has been suggested that a large proportion of the ethnic minority population in the UK is concerned about being a victim of racism and feeling vulnerable to experiences of racism may be associated with poorer health experience (Karlsen and Nazroo 2004). These aspects of quality of life can be addressed by public policy and should be a priority if the quality of extended life years is to be enhanced.

A clear understanding of what exactly is meant by mental health is also important in policy, if policies are to be effective. Lack of definition in policy development could result in a lack of policy focus. Consequently any attempts at evaluating improvement to well-being could be inconclusive/incomplete/ ill-informed. Policy developments in the area of mental health should aim to explicitly define their concept so that the success of their policies can be properly evaluated.

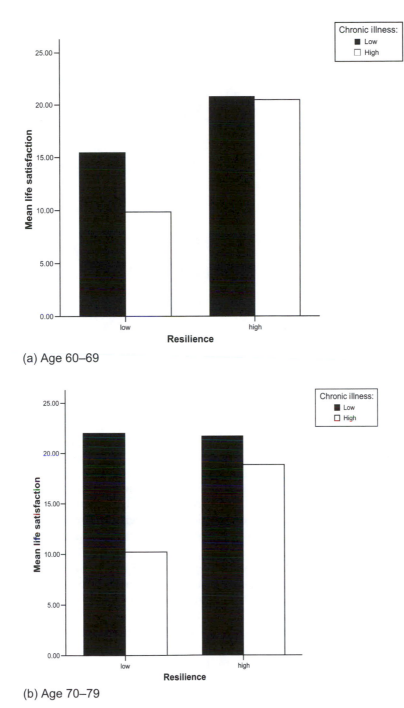

(a) Age 60–69

(b) Age 70–79

**Figure 2.5** Interaction between chronic illness and resilience by age group

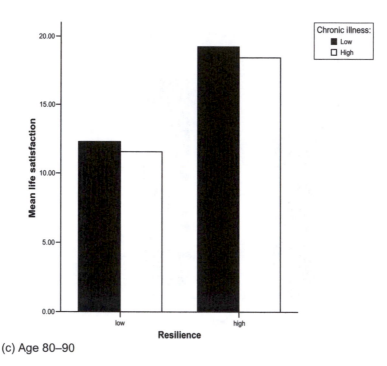

(c) Age 80–90

**Figure 2.5** Cont'd
*Source*: ESAW data

It should be stressed that there are other concepts that may be considered to represent mental health that have not been addressed here. However, this chapter has focused on some of the key concepts that have been used in ageing research – although a key limitation is that they primarily reflect a Western **ideology**. Understanding positive psychological functioning in developing countries appears to have received little attention to date, despite depression being regarded as the seventh most important cause of disease burden in low and middle income countries (WHO 2007).

This chapter has illustrated how, within the mental health framework, psychological resources such as resilience or sense of coherence can be a valuable mechanism for maintaining well-being under conditions of poor health in later life. The analyses show that although having high numbers of illnesses, over one-third of older people felt that their health was either good or excellent. This disparity has been highlighted in other research, and it has been suggested that 'older adults have higher abilities to adapt their criteria of perceived health to deteriorating objective health so that the growing number of age-associated objective health problems has only limited influence on health perception' (Pinquart 2001: 420). Maintaining favourable self-evaluations of health status is important, as self-reported health is a strong predictor of future mortality. The results of the analyses reported here suggest that psychological resilience may provide one basis for such adaptation and maintenance of life satisfaction. Importantly it shows that from the ages of 60 to 90 the participants had developed the inner capacity to deal with negative changes that are part of their ageing process, supporting the idea of 'continuity with challenge' (Atchley 1999). Such findings indicate that efforts to reduce ill health and to increase resilience would be beneficial to well-being in older age.

To conclude, the importance of good mental health and well-being to 'ageing well' cannot be emphasized enough. Public policies need to address the wide-ranging **inequalities** in later life that have a negative impact on mental well-being. Likewise those suffering from significant mental illnesses should be provided with the support and services that they deserve in their later years of life.

## Reflective questions

1   How might people from developing nations with strikingly different life-styles define mental health?
2   Consider the evidence for the determinants of mental well-being. Are these likely to be the same in developing nations?
3   How might the mental well-being of different cultures be measured or promoted?

## References

Antonovsky, A. (1987) *Unravelling the Mystery of Health.* San Francisco: Jossey-Bass.

Atchley, R. C. (1989) A continuity theory of normal aging, *The Gerontologist*, 29(2): 183–90.

Atchley, R. C. (1999) *Continuity and Adaptation in Aging.* Baltimore, MD: Johns Hopkins University Press.

Badger, T. A. (1993) Physical health impairment and depression among older adults, *Journal of Nursing Scholarship*, 25: 325–30.

Badger, T. A. (2001) Depression, psychological resources and health-related quality of life in older adults 75 and above, *Journal of Clinical Geropsychology*, (7)3: 189–200.

Ballard, C. G., Bannister, C. and Oyebode, F. (1995) Review: depression in dementia suffers, *International Journal of Geriatric Psychiatry*, 11: 507–15.

Baltes, M. M. and Baltes, P. B. (1986) *The Psychology of Control and Aging.* Hillsdale, NJ: Erlbaum.

Baltes, P. B. (1993) The aging mind: potential and limits, *The Gerontologist*, 33(5): 580–94.

Baltes, P. B. and Mayer, K. U. (1999) *The Berlin Aging Study: Aging from 70 to 100.* Cambridge: Cambridge University Press.

Baron, R. M. and Kenny, D. A. (1986) The moderator–mediator variable distinction in social psychological research: conceptual, strategic, and statistical considerations, *Journal of Personality and Social Psychology*, 51(6): 1173–82.

Bisschop, M. I., Kriegsman, D. M. W., Beekman, A. T. F. and Deeg, D. J. H. (2004) Chronic diseases and depression: the modifying role of psychosocial resources, *Social Science and Medicine*, 59: 721–33.

Bond, J. and Corner, L. (2004) *Quality of Life and Older People*. Maidenhead: Open University Press.

Bostock, Y. and Millar, C. (2003) *Older People's Perceptions of the Factors that Affect Mental Well-Being in Later Life: Final Report*. Edinburgh: NHS Health Scotland.

Bowling, A. (1991) *Measuring Health: A Review of Quality of Life Measurement Scale*. Buckingham: Open University Press.

Bowling, A. (2004) A taxonomy and overview of quality of life, in J. Brown, A. Bowling and T. Flynn (eds) *Models of Quality of Life: A Taxonomy, Overview And Systematic Review of the Literature*. Sheffield: European Forum on Population Ageing Research.

Bowling, A., Farquhar, M., Grundy, E. and Formby, J. (1993) Changes in life satisfaction over a two and a half year period among very elderly people living in London, *Social Science and Medicine*, 36(5): 641–55.

Bowling, A., Gabriel, Z., Dykes, J. et al. (2003) What people say: definitions of quality of life and its enhancement among people aged 65 and over, *International Journal of Aging and Human Development*, 56: 269–306.

Bowling, A., Grundy, E. and Farquhar, M. (1997) *Living Well into Old Age*. York: Joseph Rowntree Foundation.

Brief, A. P., Butcher, A. H., George, J. M. and Link, K. E. (1993) Integrating top–down and bottom–up theories of subjective well-being: the case of health, *Journal of Personality and Social Psychology* 64: 646–53.

Brown, J. and Flynn, T. (2004) The components of quality of life nominated by older people: a systematic review of the literature, in J. Brown, A. Bowling and T. Flynn (eds), *Models of Quality of Life: A Taxonomy, Overview and Systematic Review of the Literature*. Sheffield: European Forum on Population Ageing Research

Burholt, V., Windle, G. and Edwards, R. T. (2003) *Housing for an Ageing Population: Planning Implications: Final Report*. Bangor: Centre for Social Policy Research and Development, University of Wales.

Burnard, P., Naiyapatana, W. and Lloyd, G. (2006) Views of mental illness and mental health care in Thailand: a report of an ethnographic study, *Journal of Psychiatric and Mental Health Nursing*, 13: 742–9.

Diener, E. (1984) Subjective well-being, *Psychological Bulletin*, 95(3): 542–75.

Diener, E., and Suh, E. M. (1997) Subjective well-being and age: an international analysis, *Annual Review of Gerontology and Geriatrics*, 17: 304–24.

Diener, E., Suh, E. M., Lucas, R. E. and Smith, H. L. (1999) Subjective well-being: three decades of progress, *Psychological Bulletin*, 2: 276–302.

Diener, E., Suh, E. and Oishi, S. (1997) Recent findings on subjective well-being: *Indian Journal of Clinical Psychology*, 24: 25–41.

Eriksson, M. and Lindström, B. (2005) Antonovsky's date sense of coherence scale and the relation with health: a systematic review, *Journal of Epidemiology and Community Health*, 60: 376–81.

Ferreira, M. and Makoni, S. (2002) Towards a cultural and linguistic construction of late-life dementia in an urban African population, in S. Makoni and K. Stroeken (eds) *Ageing in Africa*. Aldershot: Ashgate.

Francis, J. and Allgar, V. (2005) Things to do, places to go: promoting mental health and well-being in later life. The findings from a call for evidence of how to promote mental health and well-being in later life – a report by Third Sector First. Available at: http://www.mhilli.org/documents/Thingstodoplacestogo-FINAL.pdf (accessed 17 Oct. 2008).

Gallo, L. C., Bogart, L. M., Vranceanu, A. and Mathews, K. A. (2005) Socioeconomic status, resources, psychological experiences and emotional responses: A test of the reserve capacity model, *Journal of Personality and Social Psychology*, 88(2): 386–99.

Gupta, S. (1992) Psychosis in Asia immigrants from the Indian sub-continent: preliminary findings from a follow-up study including survey of general practitioners, *Social Psychiatry and Psychiatric Epidemiology*, 27(5): 242–4.

Haug, M. R. and Folmar, S. J. (1986) Longevity, gender and life quality, *Journal of Health and Social Behaviour*, 27: 332–45.

Higgs, P. (1995) Citizenship and old age: the end of the road? *Ageing and Society*, 15: 535–50.

Jahoda, M. (1958) *Current Concepts of Positive Mental Health*. New York: Basic Books.

Kahana, E., Redmond, C. and Hill, G. J. et al. (1995) The effects of stress, vulnerability and appraisals on the psychological well-being of the elderly, *Research on Aging*, 17(4): 459–89.

Karlsen, S. and Nazroo, J. Y. (2004) Fear of racism and health, *Journal of Epidemiology and Community Health*, 58: 1017–18.

Knipscheer, C. P. M., Broese van Groenou, M. I., Leene, G. J. F., Beekman, A. T. F., and Deeg, D. J. H. (2000) The effects of environmental context and personal resources on depressive symptomology in older age: a test of the Lawton model, *Ageing and Society*, 20: 183–202.

Knowles, C. (1991) Afro-Caribbeans and schizophrenia: how does psychiatry deal with issues of race, culture and ethnicity? *Journal of Social Policy*, 20(2): 173–90.

Lachman, M. E. (1986) Personal control in later life: stability, change and cognitive correlates, in M. M. Baltes and P. B. Baltes (eds) *The Psychology of Control and Aging*. Hillsdale, NJ: Erlbaum.

Lachman, M. E. and Weaver, S. L. (1998) The sense of control as a moderator of social class differences in health and well-being, *Journal of Personality and Social Psychology*, 74(3): 763–73.

Landau, R. and Litwin, H. (2001) Subjective well-being among the old-old: the role of health, personality and social support, *International Journal of Ageing and Human Development*, 54(4): 265–89.

Lawton, M. P. (1983) Environment and other determinants of well-being in older people, *The Gerontologist*, 23: 134–43.

Lee, M. (2006) *Promoting Mental Health and Well-being in Later Life: A First Report from the UK Inquiry into Mental Health and Mental Well-being in Later Life*. London: Age Concern and the Mental Health Foundation.

Masten, A. S. (1999) Resilience comes of age: reflections on the past and outlook for the next generation of research, in M. D. Glantz and J. Johnson (eds) *Resilience and Development: Positive Life Adaptations. Longitudinal Research in the Social and Behavioral Sciences*. New York: Plenum Press.

McCracken, C. F. M., Boneham, M. A. and Copeland, J. R. M. (1997) Prevalence of dementia and depression among elderly people in black and ethnic minorities, *British Journal of Psychiatry*, 171: 269–73.

Morawetz, C. Ackermann, K. and Wormstall, H. (2001) Psychosocial aspects of mild cognitive impairment in the elderly, *Zeitschrift für Gerontopsychologie & Psychiatrie*, 14(3): 137–42.

Nazroo, J. Y. (1997) *The Health of Britain's Ethnic Minorities*. London: Policy Studies Institute.

O'Mahony, J. M. and Connelly, T. T. (2007) The influence of culture on immigrant women's mental health care experiences from the perspectives of health care providers, *Issues in Mental Health Nursing*, 28: 453–71.

Pearlin, L. I., Menaghan, E. G., Lieberman, M. A. and Mullan, J. T. (1981) The stress process, *Journal of Health and Social Behaviour*, 22: 337–56.

Pinquart, M. (2001) Correlates of subjective health in older adults: a meta-analysis, *Psychology and Aging*, 16(3): 414–26.

Pinquart, M. and Sörensen, S. (2001). Gender differences in self-concept and psychological well-being in old age: a meta-analysis, *Journal of Gerontology: Psychological Sciences*, 56B(4): 195–213.

Prince, M. J., Beekman, A. T. F., Deeg, D. J. H. et al. (1999) Depression symptoms in late life assessed using the EURO-D scale: effect of age, gender and marital status in 14 European countries, *British Journal of Psychiatry*, 174: 339–45.

Rutter, M. (1987) Psychosocial resilience and protective mechanisms, *American Journal of Orthopsychiatry*, 57(3): 316–31.

Rutter, M. (1995) Psychosocial adversity: risk, resilience and recovery, *Southern African Journal of Child & Adolescent*, 7(2): 75–88.

Ryff, C. D. (1989) In the eye of the beholder: views of psychological well-being among middle aged and older adults, *Psychology and Aging*, 4: 195–210.

Ryff, C. D. and Keyes, C. L. M. (1995) The structure of psychological well-being revisited, *Journal of Personality and Social Psychology*, 69(4): 719–27.

Ryff, C. D. and Singer, B. (1996) Psychological well-being: meaning, measurement and implications for psychotherapy research, *Psychotherapy and Psychosomatics*, 65: 14–23.

Sands, L. P., Ferreira, P., Steward, A. L., Brod, M. and Yaffe, K. (2004) What explains differences between dementia patients and their caregivers' ratings of patients' quality of life? *American Journal of Geriatric Psychiatry*, 13(3): 272–80.

Scottish Executive (2006) *Strategy for Scotland's Ageing Population: Omnibus Survey Findings*. Edinburgh: Scottish Executive Social Research.

Siddell, M. (1995) *Health in Old Age: Myth, Mystery and Management*. Buckingham: Open University Press.

Smith, A. (2000) *Researching Quality of Life of Older People: Concepts, Measures and Findings*. Working Paper No. 7. Keele: Centre for Social Gerontology, Keele University.

Sproston, K. and Nazroo, J. (eds) (2002) *Ethnic Minority Psychiatric Illness Rates in the Community (EMPIRIC)*. London: TSO.

Staudinger, U. M. (2000) Many reasons speak against it, yet many people feel good: the paradox of subjective well-being, *Psychologische Rundschau*, 51(4): 185–97.

Teri, L. and Wagner, A. W. (1992) Alzheimer's disease and depression, *Journal of Consulting and Clinical Psychology*, 60: 379–91.

UN (United Nations) (2001) *World Population Aging: 1950–2050*. New York: Department of Economic and Social Affairs Population Division, UN.

Wagnild, G. M. and Young, H. M. (1993) Development and psychometric evaluation of the Resilience Scale, *Journal of Nursing Measurements*, 1: 165–78.

Waite, A., Bebbington, P., Skelton-Robinson, M. and Orell, P. (2004) Life events, depression and social support in dementia, *British Journal of Clinical Psychology*, 43: 313–24.

Wells, Y. D. and Kendig, H. L. (1999) Psychological resources and successful retirement, *Australian Psychologist*, 34(2): 111–15.

Wenger, G. C., Davies, R., Shahatahmasebi, S. and Scott, A. (1996) Social isolation and loneliness in old age: review and model refinement, *Ageing and Society*, 16: 333–58.

White, A. (2007) A global projection of subjective well-being: a challenge to positive psychology? *Psychtalk* 56: 17–20. Available at: http://www.le.ac.uk/users/aw57/world/sample.html (accessed 17 Oct. 2008).

WHO (World Health Organization) (1986) *Ottawa Charter for Health Promotion: First International Conference on Health Promotion*, Ottawa, 17–21 November.

WHO (World Health Organization) (2005) *Promoting Mental Health: Concepts, Emerging Evidence, Practice*. Geneva: WHO in collaboration with the Victoria Health Foundation (VicHealth) and the University of Melbourne.

WHO (World Health Organisation) (2007) *Mental Health: A State of Well-Being*. Available at: http://www.who.int/topics/mental_health/factsheets/en/index.html (accessed 17 Oct. 2008).

Windle, G. (2006) Variations in subjective well-being: the role of psychological resilience in older age. Unpublished PhD thesis, Bangor University.

Windle, G., Markland, D. A., and Woods, B. (2008) Examination of a theoretical model of psychological resilience in older age, *Aging & Mental Health*, 12(3): 285–92.

Windle, G. and Woods, R. T. (2004) Variations in subjective well-being: the mediating role of a psychological resource, *Ageing and Society*, 24: 583–602.

Wood, V., Wylie, M. L. and Scheafor, B. (1969) An analysis of a short self-report measure of life satisfaction: correlation with rater judgements, *Journal of Gerontology*, 2: 465–9.

# 3 Theoretical perspectives on ageing and health promotion
## Sylvia Tilford

## Editor's foreword

In order to understand why or why not interventions work it is useful to have an understanding of their theoretical grounding. Theory provides the framework for effective interventions and can help to develop and position activities within our own set of values and ideologies. This chapter starts with an interesting discussion about the meaning of theory and the distinction between theory and models. It goes on to consider relevant mental health theories and models in later life, and provides a useful summary and reflections of the main theories of ageing. The values and principles underpinning health promotion theory are also explored and how these relate to mental health promotion in later life. The second part of the chapter focuses on how theory can be applied in mental health promotion and provides a number of excellent examples of theory-based mental health activities for older people.

## Introduction

Good health promotion practice is based on a number of factors of which theory, evidence and values and ideology are key ones. The importance of **evidence-based practice** is now widely accepted and there have been initiatives to support practitioners in accessing and using evidence. Arguably there has not been the same attention to theory-based practice. Overall health promotion values and **ideologies** inform the nature of practice, the kinds of evidence that are sought as a basis for it, and the theories that are used to guide practice and its evaluation. Although the main focus of this chapter is on theoretical perspectives, reference will also be made to evidence, values and ideologies. After brief introductory comments on the nature of theory, an overview of main theoretical perspectives on ageing and on health promotion will be provided. The second part of the chapter will illustrate the use of theories in selected practice examples.

## What is theory?

Theory helps us to understand the complexities of the natural and social world. A typical definition describes theory as 'an abstract set of concepts and propositions which can be applied to a variety of situations in order to explain or predict events' (National Cancer Institute 2005). This definition fits with a scientific and **positivist** paradigm where theories are developed by deduction from first principles as well as induction from empirical data, and supporting evidence is then sought. A key feature of such theories is their generalizability, a feature specific to theories in the natural sciences but also claimed for the social sciences. While some social science theories may achieve a measure of generalizability, very many do not. It has been argued that the social sciences need an alternative approach to theory provided by the **interpretivist** paradigm where theory is drawn inductively from the results of qualitative studies. Instead of prizing prediction and control, interpretivist theories focus on developing understanding and offering explanations. For example, Taraborrelli (1993) offers a theoretical model explaining three career paths to becoming a carer. While generalizability is not claimed for such theories, some transferability to similar situations can be. All theories can be amended in the light of experience or rejected when newer ones emerge offering better explanations. When this happens, the older ones may still continue to have influence. Health promotion draws on theories from both the positivist and interpretivist traditions.

Concepts and theories to support mental health promotion practice are twofold: those which assist in understanding the people with whom we are working and support analysis of issues to be addressed, and those which support the planning, implementation and evaluation of actions. This theory base is an integration of theories from different disciplines including psychology, sociology, education and social policy. In practice the selection of theories will differ according to the task in hand and ideological commitments. For example, if the primary goal of practice is behaviour change designed to lead to the prevention of illness, there are theories which are especially relevant to this. On the other hand if the goal is to empower people and promote positive mental health and to act on the social determinants of health, a different mix of theories will be relevant.

## Theories and models

These need to be distinguished. Like theories, models are aids to understanding. Some are simply visual representations and not based on theory. Theoretical models, on the other hand, represent the elements of a specific theory or a combination of theories. Macdonald and Hara's (Macdonald 2006: 22) ten element map of mental health and its promotion is a relevant example (see Figure 3.1). This belongs to a general class of ecological models which integrate micro, meso and macro elements. A further group of models, the Health Belief Model, Theory of Planned Behaviour and Health Action Model present factors which influence health-related decision-making. Where individual theoretical concepts are concerned, some, such as self-efficacy, appear in a number of theories and models, while others may be confined to a single theory.

There are various ways that mental health promotion theories can be categorized, for example:

1 According to level of analysis ranging from the individual (micro-level determinants) to family and community (**meso-level determinants**) through to societal (macro-level determinants); or combinations of these levels as in ecological models

2 In relation to the area of activity: e.g. theories for the analysis of situations requiring action versus theories used to inform planning and implementation of activities. Assigning theories to categories is not always clear-cut and a number of theories may be drawn on in both analysis and planning (see Box 3.1).

Space precludes a detailed discussion of all concepts and theories listed in Box 3.1 some of which are considered elsewhere in the book. Selected theories will be discussed briefly either in this section or in the second part of the chapter when they form the framework for specific programmes. Some additional theories will also be included in later chapters. Details of common theories and models and their constituent concepts can be found in *Theory at a Glance* (National Cancer Institute 2005), *Theory in a Nutshell* (Nutbeam and Harris 2004) and in general health promotion texts (Naidoo and Wills 2000; Tones and Tilford 2001; Tones and Green 2004).

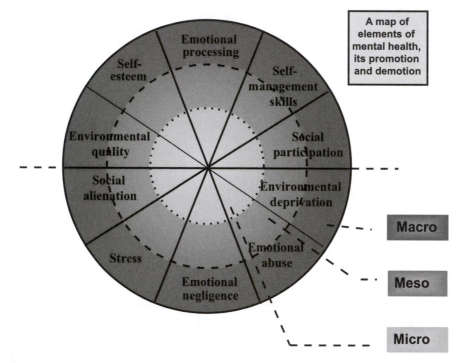

**Figure 3.1** Macdonald and O'Hara's ten element map
*Source*: Macdonald (2006: 22)

---

**Box 3.1** Theories and models for mental health promotion in later life

| ANALYSIS OF ISSUES | IMPLEMENTATION & EVALUATION |
|---|---|
| **Concepts** | **Concepts** |
| Ageing, ageism, identity, efficiency, esteem, stigma, discrimination, equity and inequality, gender, ethnicity, resilience, empowerment, salutogenesis, social capital, loneliness, cohesion | Sustainability, gender, ethnicity, ageism, ethics, evidence, effectiveness, efficiency |
| **Models and theories** | **Models and theories** |
| Mental health and mental health promotion | Communication and education |
| Lifespan development | Behaviour change |
| Individual health decision-making | Social learning |
| Ageing | Policy development |
| Psychosocial transitions and change | Communication of innovations |
| | Social networks theory |
| | Management of change |
| | Programme planning |
| | Evaluation theory |

---

## Selected theories and models

This section provides a brief introduction to three areas of theory: perspectives on ageing; perspectives on health promotion practice; and perspectives on evaluation. These have relevance to discussion in a number of chapters.

### Perspectives on ageing

Many theories have been developed to explain the nature of ageing and the relationship of the later years to the lifespan, originating from a number of disciplines including psychology and sociology. Theories differ in their conceptions of the later years and of the progression through life. Many have arisen predominantly from Western contexts and it is essential to consider the extent to which they offer partial explanations. It is also important to consider the relative influence of the differing theories and to question the extent to which they match with lay perspectives (Rogers and Pilgrim 1997; Bostock and Millar 2003). Theories can be divided into the biological and the socio-psychological. We will not consider the biological theories beyond noting that they can be divided into the genetic and non-genetic and that there is currently no one accepted theory of biological ageing. Many early psychological theories started from a consideration of childhood and conceived of growth and development as an upward progression through stages from childhood to adulthood, a plateau phase, followed by decline. Relatively little attention was paid to the adult period, even less to the later years and the conception offered of them was somewhat negative. A stage-based theory which did address the full lifespan was that of Erikson (1963) where the later years were understood in the context of preceding life phases, each of which has psychosocial tasks to be overcome in order to cope with the next phases. Contemporary lifespan psychology adopts a less **deterministic** and less individualistic approach proposing that: the potential for development crosses the lifespan; there is no predetermined route that development does or should take; there are differing strands within development; and there should be a person-in-environment focus.

A small selection of social science theories on ageing is presented in Box 3.2. For a detailed consideration of theory development on ageing and a critique of individual theories readers are referred to Marcoen et al. (2007) and Phillipson and Baars (2007).

---

## Box 3.2 Theories of ageing

*Disengagement theory:* This was developed by Cumming and Henry (1961) and it describes ageing as an inevitable process in which people disengage from society with a loss of roles especially validated by society, have restricted social contacts, and have reduced commitment to some social norms. The process is conceptualized as good for older people themselves as well as for society and as a **functionalist theory** helps to explain the transfer of power between generations.

*Activity theory:* Havighurst and Albrecht (1953) proposed that successful ageing involves the preservation for as long as possible of the attitudes and activities of the middle years. Self-identity is based on the number and types of roles held by individuals. When some activities and roles are surrendered, substitute ones need to be taken on to maintain self-esteem.

*Continuity theory:* This theory (Atchley 1989) claims that older adults, after retiring from paid work, try to maintain stability in the lifestyle which has been developed earlier and a sense of self-esteem and other values. Reflection on past experience and setting goals for the future are key processes. Individuals, it is proposed, need to manage change in a positive and empowering way.

*Age stratification theory:* This theory (Riley 1988) introduced the influence of social structure on individual ageing. People of the same ages form cohorts – or age strata – who share historical experiences as well as individual ones. Successive strata of 70-year-olds will have had different historical experiences.

*Structured dependency theory*: It is societal structures which make older people dependent. Because of retirement age requirements they have to leave the workforce and are supported in doing so by the existence of pensions, which are mostly limited. The respect which they receive from society, as non-workers, is reduced. Societal stereotypes of ageing – largely negative – increase the separation of older people (Wilson 2000: 12).

*Labelling theory*: This is derived from sociology of deviance theory. Old age is seen as a deviant condition. People define themselves according to how others react and their behaviour in later life is, therefore, socially determined by the norms of society (Becker 1963).

*Exchange theory:* This theory focuses on the exchange of material and non-material goods and services in societies. People pursue common goals and enter into social relationships which entail costs. Efforts are made to maximize gains and minimize costs. As people get older their power in the processes of social exchange diminishes and they can become powerless, passive and compliant (Dowd 1975).

*Social interactionist (constructionist) theory:* This is based on the work of Mead (1934) and Berger and Luckman (1966). For the individual, ageing is not passively determined by biological, psychological or sociological processes, but is the product of individuals' objective and subjective experiences as they interact with the social world. In society as a whole the concept of ageing is a product of social interactions where some have greater power than others to influence ideas.

*Political economy theory:* This theory takes into consideration the divisions between older people arising from class, gender, ethnicity and other bases of inequality. It builds on structured dependency theory and addresses the differential effects of retirement on older people according to prior socio-economic and other bases of inequality (Phillipson and Baars 2007).

## Reflections of theories of ageing

Briefly, the theories outlined, together with others, differ in the weight they place on individual as opposed to societal explanations for ageing, the extent to which they are positive or negative about ageing and the degree to which they are deterministic. In general there has been some shift from theorizing about ageing as essentially a negative experience for those involved, and a problem for societies, towards more positive conceptions. Although research support has been offered for the various theories, many have also been challenged on the basis of other research or on contextual evidence. For example, disengagement theory, an early theory, has been particularly challenged as being as positivist and determinist. In many cultures people do leave the formal workforce at particular ages and most do disengage from many, if not all, of the activities that this entailed. This can have consequences for self-esteem where this has been strongly influenced by occupation. In Bostock and Miller's (2003) interviews there were comments about 'being on the scrap heap' a phrase that is widely heard. Disengagement from occupational roles in later life is not, however, universal and also does not necessarily symbolize general disengagement as presented in the theory. Engagement with occupational roles is frequently replaced by new or enhanced alternatives which are highly valued – in voluntary work, occupationally related activity, grandparenting, and so on. The activity model, another early theory, is also prescriptive about the ageing process and the transition between middle and later years although the theory is less deterministic. Age stratification theory, although recognizing the similarities shared by age cohorts, has been criticized for its limited emphasis on individual differences.

The importance of theories of ageing derived from non-Western cultures has been recognized as earlier assumptions about the universal relevance of Western generated theory have been challenged (Giddens 1989: 597). As societies, such as in the UK, become increasingly multicultural, the relevance of existing theories of ageing for understanding minority elders has to be reassessed. Claims that ageing in non-Western 'traditional' societies has more positive connotations and that older people are accorded greater respect and status in these societies have also to be interrogated. Such idealized conceptions can obscure the differences between and across such societies related to gender, ethnicity and caste. More generally, the existence of globalization leads to the need to theorize further about ageing world-wide (see, for example, Aboderin 2004).

Can any one theory adequately represent ageing in contemporary society across cultures? Furthermore do we even want one single theory? In an era of postmodernism there has been a move away from the importance of generating universal positivist theories, a greater acceptance of theories from non-positivist traditions and a readiness to identify and respect lay theories, often close to interpretivist ones. As Wilson (2000: 12) has said: 'A theory that could accommodate the diverse views of elders themselves would have the edge over a theory that simply told them what they were from an academic perspective.' Davies, in noting the genesis of most theories of ageing in academic contexts and probably from younger academics, has also emphasized (National Council for the Elderly 1994: 10) the need for older people themselves to be involved in the development of theories of ageing and in tackling ageism.

While accepting that no single theory can adequately explain ageing, the various theories available can be useful if drawn on to aid understanding and support actions but do not become self-fulfilling prophecies (National Council for the Elderly 1994). Furthermore, while theories may conflict logically (Wilson 2000: 11), they often make sense to individual elders as representations of different aspects of their lives. Although we may not wish, therefore, to pursue a quest for a single theory we can suggest the kinds of theoretical models of ageing that would be useful as frameworks for mental health promotion. These would recognize the variety of life experiences within specific cultural contexts of people in later years, and the social pressures and expectations that provide the context for their lives. Theories would also operate from a positive rather than negative conception of older people, would be in tune with core ideas of health promotion, and would take into consideration gender and ethnicity. In developing such models older people's theorizing would be taken into account. Theory should also recognize the differences that can exist for people in the fourth age when compared with the third age, with the former having received less consideration than the latter in theoretical work (Phillipson and Baars 2007: 60).

# Theoretical positions on mental health promotion practice

Health promotion is not practised in accordance with one agreed set of goals and processes. There are alternative approaches informed by sets of values or ideological positions with differing goals. These have been categorized in a variety of ways (see, for example, Beattie 1991; Naidoo and Wills 2000; Tones and Tilford 2001; Tones and Green 2004). Whether all categorizations should be described as analytical and theoretical as opposed to descriptive is open to discussion. We will draw on two typologies which can be classed as analytical. Beattie's 2 × 2 (1991) model is particularly useful for helping to locate the bases of individual practice. It distinguishes the types of mental health promotion intervention on a scale from fully negotiated through to professionally determined, and the focus of practice ranging from the individual to the collective. An illustration of this model with reference to promoting mental health in later life is provided in Figure 3.2.

If we are seeking to work in mental health promotion in ways that take clients' views into consideration, we are likely to focus on the personal counselling and community development quadrants of Beattie's model complemented by legislative action where necessary. There may be times where activity within the health persuasion quadrant is justified – when people cannot, for physical or mental reasons, engage in a personal counselling approach or where they specifically demand and

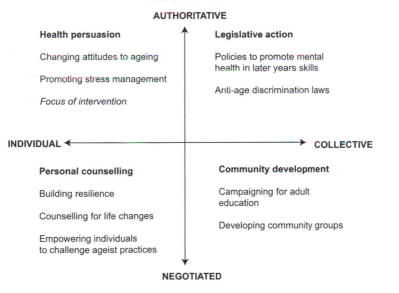

**Figure 3.2**  Beattie's model of health promotion applied to mental health in later life

agree to work informed by a preventive approach. It remains the case that much mental health promotion activity does sit within the health persuasion quadrant, reflecting widespread adherence to this approach.

## Prevention versus empowerment

A simpler distinction can be made between a preventive medical model and an empowerment model, drawing on the various categorizations developed over the years by Tones (in Tones and Tilford 2001; Tones and Green 2004). The preventive model, derived from the classic medical model, conceptualizes health promotion as a process designed to secure changes in behaviours which are linked to health outcomes. The methods used are determined by professionals and may either address behaviours directly or those factors such as knowledge, beliefs and attitudes which are related to behaviours. This model closely matches the persuasion quadrant in the Beattie model. A practice example would be a programme for care home residents designed to increase physical activity in order to enhance mental health, without reference to resident needs and preferences or involving their participation in planning the programme. Within mental health promotion this approach can also be called a risk reduction model (Mrazek and Haggerty 1994) and is the basis for a number of programmes. An empowerment approach, on the other hand, has as its key goal the empowerment of individuals or groups to be able to take health-related decisions. Activities are based on participatory needs assessment and can include facilitation of knowledge gain, development of critical literacy skills, self-efficacy and self-esteem, resilience, counselling and advocacy skills. The competence enhancement model, discussed in detail by Barry (2001) is closely related to the empowerment model. It is an extension of the risk reduction model, considers individuals and communities within the wider socio-cultural context and emphasizes the key role of empowerment.

The approach adopted can be taken solely on ideological grounds but in practice is also likely to be influenced by:

1   The particular preferences and the capacities of the people with whom work is being undertaken.
2   Contextual factors which make some types of practice difficult. For example, resources are not available to support a full empowerment approach or workers are expected to account for their practice in behaviour change or health outcome terms.

## Evaluation theory

Mental health promotion programmes require some critical reflection on their processes and outcomes to check effectiveness and that resources have been wisely used and to ensure that there has been no negative impact on the participants. Evaluation is the assessment of a programme against its objectives in order to identify ways of improving it. The findings from evaluation studies and other research studies help to build the evidence base for practice. There are distinctive theoretical perspectives on evaluation which reflect alternative views on what counts as good evidence and the ways that this should be acquired as well as assumptions about the relationship between evaluators and the participants in a programme. These, again, can be divided into positivist and interpretivist theories. For positivists, greatest weight is given to quantitative evidence gained from evaluating programmes in accordance with experimental designs, in other words, **randomized controlled trials** (**RCTs**) or other studies high on the **hierarchy of evidence**. Many health promotion programmes are not amenable to such styles of evaluation. Importantly, for many health promoters, they are in conflict with the core value of health promotion which emphasizes the involvement of programme participants in evaluation rather than submitting to processes defined by others.

The interpretivist model of evaluation mainly uses methods which generate qualitative data and may include greater involvement of programme participants in decisions about the nature and process of evaluation, in data analysis and in writing up the findings. A further specific model of evaluation informed by realist theory is described as realistic or theory-based evaluation (Pawson and Tilley 1997). It is increasingly being used to evaluate complex health promotion programmes. The approach seeks to identify what works, for whom, and in what circumstances, and has been used in evaluating Health Action Zone and Sure Start programmes in the UK.

There have been lively debates across health promotion about how evaluation should be undertaken and the kinds of evidence that should be generated. If published reports of mental health promotion studies are examined, the evidence most frequently reported comes from psychological-type interventions, evaluated by RCTs or alternative strong designs. According to Secker (1998), the consequence is that more of the same types of interventions are carried out because they are supported by the published evidence. It can be argued that some simple health promotion actions such as information and communication can be evaluated by use of an RCT without there being serious ethical or other concerns. In general, however, holistic multi- component programmes need different evaluation approaches. Overall there is broad support for the adoption of methods drawn from the differing paradigms of evaluation in order to generate a comprehensive picture of the effectiveness and process of programmes.

## Application of theory to mental health promotion from a lay perspective of mental health and well-being

Mental health promotion practice may be based on an idea of what works, the published evidence base, values, a directive from others, efforts to be innovative, funding constraints or it can be based on theory. Usually it is some combination of these factors, but as Caplan and Holland (1990: 12) said: 'effective practice in health promotion depends on good theory'. The theories drawn on will depend on the health promotion issue to be addressed and the stage of the process and single theories or various combinations can be used. The importance of theory for practice has been summarized (National Cancer Institute 2005; see also Box 3.3). Having stressed this importance, it has to be acknowledged that in many reports of practice, theory is not mentioned explicitly and it is not easy to detect implicit use. Cattan (2006), commenting on a systematic review of evaluations of mental health promotion activities with older people, noted that only a proportion appeared to be theory based with one-third making no mention of theory. Where the theoretical basis was stated, some form of behavioural theory was most frequently used. Studies that meet criteria for inclusion in systematic reviews are not fully representative. For example, community-generated activities which conform to principles of empowerment and community development are typically not evaluated in ways that lead them to be selected for systematic reviews. If we look at evaluations of mental health promotion activities appearing in unpublished as well as published literature, we may expect to find evidence of the use of a wider range of theories.

---

**Box 3.3** How theory helps in planning effective programmes

- Provides tools for moving beyond intuition.
- Helps in standing back and considering the larger picture.
- Grounding interventions in theory can lead to creative practice.
- Consistent with evidence-based practice.
- Provides a road map for studying problems, developing appropriate interventions and evaluating successes.
- Helps to explain the dynamics of health behaviours, the influences on them and the processes for change.
- Helps in identifying indicators for use evaluations.
  (After National Cancer Institute 2005)

---

## Examples of theory-based mental health projects for people in later years

The aim in this section is to describe a small selection of theory-based activities linked to the perspectives on mental health which emerged from the Scottish survey discussed in earlier chapters (Bostock and Millar 2003). To do this it was necessary to identify programmes that have done more than draw on well-tested psychological models of behaviour change. In general, it is more difficult to find examples of theory-based programmes designed for people in later years than it is for other age groups. This may reflect the actual level of activity and/or fewer publication opportunities. If there is less activity designed for people in later years than for younger age groups, this is not necessarily problematic. If people do not wish to be identified and labelled as older, they may prefer programmes designed for adults in general. A lack of specific programmes may, however, mean that needs are not being met fully. Connell (1999), moreover, reminds us of the diversity of people who are over 60 which needs to be reflected in the programmes being planned.

## Empowerment

Earlier we have discussed the importance of an empowerment approach to health promotion. One programme, the Older Women's Network (OWN), which applied empowerment theory in a community setting is a good starting point (Onyx and Benton 1995). OWN was a grassroots movement set up in the 1980s, directed by women themselves to provide a means through which they could meet others with similar interests and challenge stereotyped images. Its activities included activity sessions for women themselves and provision of advice to governments. It fulfilled the theoretical criteria for community development, with women:

- identifying their own needs;
- identifying constraints;
- determining alternative courses of action;
- drawing on appropriate resources from within OWN or from elsewhere;
- carrying out actions involving participation of members and evaluation.

As Onyx and Benton (1995: 56) explain: 'The women are proactive in seeking to influence others, locating additional resources to do so in developing their skills and knowledge, self confidence and mutual support. They are clearly empowering themselves. In the process they explicitly negate the image of the helpless, hapless, useless old woman.'

In the Scottish survey (Bostock and Millar 2003) one of the three reported key barriers to mental health was fear of loss of independence, which relates to the concepts of autonomy and empowerment. Heathcote (2000), in qualitative research with older people in the UK and Italy, identified the retention of autonomy as a dominant emergent theme. She also elicited views from professionals and from volunteers working with older people. On the basis of findings, a health education handbook was developed offering lifeskills strategies for empowerment focused on developing positive self-image, social ease and feelings of belongingness. The activities included: expressive arts and physical, social and other educative activities. An important observation was made on professionals' use of theory. Prior to project involvement they were not working to a conscious or explicit model of lifeskills development although they had implicitly assumed a relationship between such development and well-being, health, social inclusion, autonomy and empowerment.

## *Change and transitions*

Coping with change is necessary at all ages but a number of major changes can affect later years and have been recognized as barriers to mental health (Bostock and Millar 2003). Various theoretical accounts of the process of change and coping with it have been drawn from major life changes (Benoliel 1999). A widely used model (Figure 3.3) represents the reaction and adaptation to change as a staged process with levels of mood varying across stages (Adams et al. 1976; Sugarman 1986).

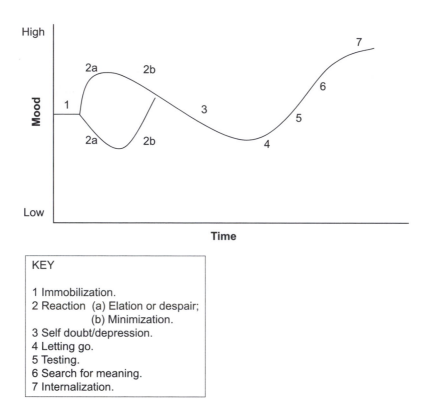

**Figure 3.3** The 7-phase model of stages accompanying transitions
*Source*: Adapted from Hopson (1981); Sugarman (1986)

While many people will follow the type of progression shown in response to a major change, it should not be assumed that all will or should. Responses can vary according to the nature of change, individuals' perceptions of it and contextual factors. While the model helps in recognizing the complexity of responses to a change, it needs to be used with care. Programmes to support coping with change can be initiated in anticipation of changes as well as during the process. An example of the former was a two-year pilot programme of eight projects designed to reach people at times of transition. It aimed to engage clients between 50–65 years and empower them through pre-retirement health advice and services (Secker et al. 2005). Activities varied across the projects and included short pre-retirement courses, provision of advice by peer educators and health checks. The programme offered an example of evaluation using a theories of change approach examining the 'theories' adopted by each project in relation to the impact on clients. All projects included focus on the concepts of client engagement, empowerment and social activity.

## Adult education

Participation in adult education has been linked to mental health gains (Schuller et al. 2001; Swindell 2002). The links between creativity and health in adult education for older people have also been examined by Bennetts et al. (2005) and they have identified questions for research about the kinds of creative and educational interventions which will impact on the lives of older people's health and well-being, and their social relationships, participation in the community, self-identity, and learning and skills. One of the best known initiatives for older people is the University of the Third Age (U3A), informed by a humanistic philosophy and commitment to life-long learning. Groups, organized by members, for members, offer varied opportunities for participants to share their knowledge, skills and experience, and to achieve new learning in informal friendly atmospheres. The costs to members are very low as all facilitators of activities work on a no-fee basis. Participation can be biased towards those who are white, middle class and with greater previous educational experience. While efforts to widen participation undoubtedly occur, the barriers to participation in learning are not easily overcome for many older adults.

## Health-related behaviours

Behaviour change is a goal of some mental health promotion activity and central, as already noted, to the use of a preventive model. It can also be a goal for advocates of an empowerment model if behaviours are negotiated with those concerned, and appropriate methods are used. Several theoretical models conceptualize the factors that influence individual health behaviours and can be used in planning behavioural change activities. The oldest, and one of the most widely used, is the Health Belief Model. Developed initially with reference to the adoption of immunizations and related health behaviours, it has been applied widely to physical health behaviours which, as noted, can also influence mental health. The model was applied in a study of beliefs and attitudes of older people towards influenza and vaccination in Greece (Raftopoulos 2007). He reported that the findings demonstrated the appropriateness of the Health Belief Model as a theoretical framework for understanding uptake and planning interventions. A further model which has been widely used in health promotion is the Theory of Planned Behaviour, although no published example of an application to mental health in older people has been identified.

A third model is the Transtheoretical Model and Stages of Change (Prochaska et al. 2002). The adoption of a behaviour is conceived as a cyclical process incorporating a number of stages: precontemplation; contemplation; preparation for change; action; and maintenance. Movement through the stages is influenced by self-efficacy, and a number of processes support the progression. People may access the cycle at various stages and may relapse a number of times before finally maintaining a new behaviour. The model was used as the basis of a physical health programme on exercise and nutrition for older people in the USA (Clark et al. 2002). Primary outcomes were to increase exercise and fruit/vegetable consumption, with the secondary outcomes of improved physical functioning and overall health. According to the authors, this model was chosen for various reasons including the fact that interventions based on it have outperformed best practice interventions and it had been successfully applied to exercise in older adults. Although widely adopted it should also be noted that there have been criticisms of the model and its application, based on reviews of research evidence (Whitelaw et al 2000; Adams and White 2005). Adams and White examined physical activity interventions and concluded that there was a lack of evidence of the effectiveness of stage-based interventions, and suggested a number of reasons for this related to the model itself and to the complexity of physical activity behaviours.

## Back to empowerment

Finally, a small project which brings together a number of theoretical ideas – empowerment, creativity, communication and values pertaining to professional practice. The project Empowerment Through Creativity followed a request for Bangladeshi older women in a UK city to participate in developing visual health education materials for the wider community of Bangladeshi women. A participatory, collaborative approach was adopted. Evaluation revealed that the workshops were an empowering experience through provision of a financial incentive, encouraging the learning of new skills and enhancing self-efficacy, increasing self-confidence, raising self-esteem and developing shared goals and teamwork. The project led to the development of practical guidelines for organizing similar projects (Fawbert 1999).

Later chapters in the book will refer to other mental health promotion activities and they may apply further theories not specifically illustrated in this section.

# Conclusions

Theorizing about the process of ageing is an ongoing project. Awareness of these theories is necessary in order to identify the influences they have had on mental health promotion activities with people in their later years. The theoretical basis of mental health promotion also continues to develop. Practice needs to be informed by theory, evidence and values, together with other general or specific factors. Practitioners report the use of theory in programme planning (Jones and Donovan 2004), although they are aware of more theories than they actually use. Published accounts of mental health promotion frequently omit an adequate consideration of theory. The importance of lay theorizing about ageing and mental health promotion has been noted. Where involvement in programme design and delivery is concerned, Seymour and Gale (2004) concluded in *Literature and Policy Review for the Joint Inquiry into Mental Health and Well-being in Later Life* that the most conspicuous omission from the published literature was any sense that people in later life had any input into these processes. Older people are most likely to be involved in those programmes which they themselves actually initiate, which address their individual needs, or which are directed towards social action and influencing policy-makers. These are not necessarily set up with explicit mental health goals, but where evaluated, the outcomes measured included those that were mental health related. Such programmes can be informed by various theories, implicit or explicit, but empowerment theory of some kind is often identifiable. To conclude, *Theory at a Glance* (National Cancer Institute 2005) includes a number of quotations from practitioners which highlight the importance of theory:

> Theory is different from most of the tools I use in my work. It's more abstract but that can be a plus too. A solid grounding in a handful of theories goes a long way towards helping me to think through why I approach a health problem the way I do.

> By translating concepts from theory into real-world terms, I can get my staff and community volunteers to take a closer look at why we're conducting programmes the way we do, and how they can succeed and fail.

## Reflective questions

1　In professional and lay discussions about older people, what theories of ageing can you hear reflected?
2　What health promotion theories do you currently use in your practice and why?
3　How does theory interact with other factors in deciding on practice?
4　If you map your activities on the Beattie model, what do you notice?
5　What approach(es) to mental health promotion practice do you prefer? Are there constraints on adopting your preference(s)?
6　How can older people be involved in deciding on the nature of mental health promotion activities and their evaluation?

## References

Aboderin, I. (2004) *Intergenerational Family Support and Old Age Economic Security in Ghana*. London: Zed Books.

Adams, J., Hayes, J. and Hopson, B. (1976) *Understanding and Managing Personal Change*. London: Martin Robertson.

Adams, J. and White, M. (2005) Why don't stage based activity promotion interventions work?, *Health Education Research*, 20(2): 237–43.

Atchley, R. (1989) A continuity theory of normal ageing, *Gerontologist*, 11: 13–17.

Barry, M. (2001) Promoting positive mental health: theoretical frameworks for practice, *International Journal of Mental Health Promotion*, 3(1): 25–32.

Beattie, A. (1991) Knowledge and social control in health promotion: a test case of social theory and social policy, in J. Gabe, M. Calnan and M. Bury (eds), *Sociology of the Health Service*. London: Routledge.

Becker, H. (1963) *The Outsiders*. New York: Free Press.

Bennetts, C., Holden, C. and Postlethwaite, K. (2005) A position paper: creativity, older people and health, *International Journal of Health Promotion and Education*, 43(4): 125–30.

Benoliel, J. Q. (1999) Loss and bereavement: perspectives, theories, challenges, *Canadian Journal of Nursing Research*, 30(4): 263–72.

Berger, P. and Luckman, T. (1966) *The Social Construction of Reality*. New York: Doubleday.

Bostock, Y. and Millar, C. (2003) *Older People's Perceptions of the Factors that Affect Mental Well-being in Later Life*. Edinburgh: NHS Health Scotland.

Caplan, R. and Holland, R. (1990) Rethinking health education theory, *Journal of Health Education*, 49(1): 10–12.

Cattan, M. (2006) Older people: the retirement years (65–80 years and 80+ years), in M. Cattan and S. Tilford (eds), *Mental Health Promotion: A Lifespan Approach*. Maidenhead: Open University Press/McGraw-Hill Education.

Clark, P. G., Nigg, C. R., Greene, G. et al. (2002) The study of exercise and nutrition in older Rhode Islanders (SENIORS): translating theory into research, *Health Education Research*, 17(5): 552–61.

Connell, C. (1999) Older adults in health education research: some recommendations, *Health Education Research*, 14(3): 427–31.

Cumming, E. and Henry, W. (1961) *Growing Old*. New York: Basic Books.

Dowd, J. J. (1975) Aging as exchange: a preface to theory, *Journal of Gerontology*, 30: 584–94.

Eriksen, E. H. (1963) *Childhood and Society*, 2nd edn. New York: W.W. Norton.

Fawbert, S. (1999) Empowerment through creativity: a community development approach to developing health education materials. Unpublished MSc dissertation, Leeds Metropolitan University.

Giddens, A. (1989) *Sociology*. Oxford: Polity Press.

Havighurst, R. J. and Albrecht, R. (1953) *Older People*. London: Longman.

Heathcote, G. (2000) Autonomy, health and ageing: transnational perspective, *Health Education Research*, 15(1): 13–24.

Jones, S. C. and Donovan, R. J. (2004) Does theory inform practice in Australia? *Health Education Research*, 19(1): 1–14.

Macdonald, G. (2006) What is mental health?, in M. Cattan and S. Tilford (eds), *Mental Health Promotion: A Lifespan Approach*. Maidenhead: Open University Press/ McGraw-Hill Education.

Marcoen, A., Coleman, P. G. and O'Hanlon, A. (2007) Psychological ageing, in J. Bond., S. Peace., F. Dittman-Kohli and G. Westerhoff (eds), *Ageing in Society: European Perspectives*. London: Sage Publications.

Mead, G. H. (1934) *Mind, Self and Society*. Chicago: University of Chicago Press.

Mrazek, P. J. and Haggerty, R. J. (eds) (1994) *Reducing Risks for Mental Disorders: Frontiers for Preventive Intervention Research*. Washington, DC: National Academic Press.

Naidoo, J. and Wills, J. (2000) *Health Promotion: Foundations for Practice*, 2nd edn. Edinburgh: Bailliere-Tindall.

National Cancer Institute (2005) *Theory at a Glance*. Available at: http:// www.cancer.gov/cancerinformation/theory-at-a-glance (Accessed 14 Feb. 2008).

National Council for the Elderly (1994) *Theories of Ageing and Attitudes to Ageing in Ireland*. Dublin: National Council for the Elderly.

Nutbeam, D. and Harris, E. (2004) *Theory in a Nutshell*, 2nd edn. Sydney: McGraw-Hill.

Onyx, J. and Benton, P. (1995) Empowerment and ageing: towards honoured places for crones and sages, in G. Craig and M. Mayo (eds), *Community Empowerment*. London: Zed Books.

Pawson, R. and Tilley, N. (1997) *Realistic Evaluation*. London: Sage Publications.

Phillipson, C. and Baars, J. (2007) Social theory and social ageing, in J. Bond, S. Peace, F. Dittman-Kohli and G. Westerhof (eds) *Ageing in Society: European Perspectives on Gerontology*. London: Sage Publications.

Prochaska, J. O., Redding, C. A. and Evers, K. E. (2002) The transtheoretical model and stages of change, in K. Glanz, B. K. Rimer and F. M. Lucas (eds) *Health Behaviour and Health Education*, 3rd edn. San Francisco: Jossey-Bass.

Raftopoulos, V. (2007) Beliefs, knowledge and attitudes of community dwelling Greek elders towards influenza and pneumococcal vaccination, *The Internet Journal of Epidemiology*, 4: 1–9.

Riley, M. W. (1998) Successful aging, *Gerontologist*, 38(2): 151.

Rogers, A. and Pilgrim, D. (1997) The contribution of lay understanding to the understanding and promotion of mental health, *Journal of Mental Health*, 6(1): 23–35.

Schuller, T., Bynner, J., Green, A. et al. (2001) *Modelling and Measuring the Wider Benefits of Learning*. The Wider Benefits of Learning Papers No. 1. London: The Institute of Education.

Secker, J. (1998) Current conceptualisations of mental health and mental health promotion, *Health Education Research*, 13(1): 57–66.

Secker, J., Bowers, H., Webb, D. and Llanes, M. (2005) Theories of change: what works in improving health in mid-life, *Health Education Research*, 20(4): 392–401.

Seymour, L. and Gale, E. (2004) *Literature and Policy Review for the Joint Inquiry into Mental Health and Well-being in Later Life*. London: Age Concern and the Mental Health Foundation. Also available at: www.mentality.org.uk

Sugarman, L. (1986) *Lifespan Development: Concepts, Theories and Interventions*. London: Methuen.

Swindell, R. (2002) U3A Online: a virtual university of the third age for isolated older people, *International Journal of Lifelong Education*, 15: 85–93.

Taraborrelli, P. (1993) Becoming a carer, in N. Gilbert (ed.), *Researching Social Life*. London: Sage Publications.

Tones, K. and Green, J. (2004) *Health Promotion: Planning and Strategies*. London: Sage Publications.

Tones, K. and Tilford, S. (2001) *Health Promotion: Effectiveness, Efficiency and Equity*, 3rd edn. Cheltenham: Nelson-Thornes.

Whitelaw, S., Baldwin, S., Bunton, R. and Flynn, D. (2000) The status of evidence and outcomes in stages of change research, *Health Education Research*, 15(6): 707–18.

Wilson, G. (2000) *Understanding Old Age: Critical and Global Perspectives*. London: Sage Publications.

# 4 Policy and practice in the promotion of mental health and well-being in later life
Jill Manthorpe and Steve Iliffe

## Editor's foreword

This chapter provides the critical link between the previous chapters and the ensuing four chapters by exploring what it is that drives mental health promotion, in other words, what the approaches are that are utilized to promote older people's mental health. The authors do this by considering policy and practice at three levels: primary, secondary and tertiary. In each section the relevant factors that affect older people's mental health and the policy implications are discussed and examples of evidence-based practice and current policy are provided. Importantly, both mental health service issues and the wider determinants of mental health as relating to older people are considered.

## Introduction

There is a gloominess about mental health in later life, fuelled on the one hand by epidemiological evidence of a worldwide rise in the prevalence of mental health problems, and on the other hand by the fear that current cohorts of young and middle-aged adults will be less robust and will have worse mental health in later life than past generations. Such gloom affects policy and practice alike. Taking this gloominess at face value forces us to ask to what extent mental wellness can be promoted and mental ill health can be prevented by early modification of social, educational and work environments (the impact of policy), or by individual or group psychological interventions (the question of **primary prevention** in practice). We also need to know to what extent impaired mental well-being can be restored and sustained. This restoration can take the form of **secondary level interventions** with semi-permanent effects (or in medical terms 'cure'), temporary renewal of wellbeing (**tertiary level intervention**), or stabilization of mental health and maximization of well-being, albeit at a level different from the individual's previous state.

In this chapter we will try to answer these questions by drawing on evidence and experience of policy and practice in England, starting with the promotion of mental wellness by the nurturing of protective social relationships, roles and individual coping strategies for dealing with adversity. We will use socio-medical models to illustrate the complexity of factors that sustain or undermine mental wellness. To avoid the cliché that wellness is more than the absence of illness, we will focus on precisely how mental illness is a dislocation or detachment of the individual from their lived social experiences of well-being. This detachment is a quantitatively different experience in later compared with earlier life for most people, primarily because of the accumulation of challenges and demands that arise from ageing. By ageing we mean both the position of older people in society and the changes of ageing that their bodies are undergoing. The understanding that we use here is that of mental wellness and illness being forms of ability and disability, with the latter defined as the gap between environmental demand and personal capabilities. In addition, an epidemiological model will be used to try to explain the huge variability in the susceptibility of older people to the factors that undermine mental well-being, and to demonstrate how a multiplicity of approaches to secondary and tertiary intervention should be considered. Finally, we will review individualized responses of the kind available to practitioners, as forms of tertiary and quaternary intervention.

## Primary intervention: coping strategies and mental health

There are many theories about the sources of mental well-being, emotional robustness and psychological resilience, and many facts that support or negate them. Most of these theories emphasize the origins of mental wellness and mental illness in the experiences of early life. Some combination of factors – personality, childhood traumas, poverty, and emotional deprivation – makes individuals vulnerable to mental ill health. Conversely, psychological wellness is presumed to arise out of consistently supportive relationships in early life that promote a strong sense of self-worth and self-efficacy. Both robustness and vulnerability persist throughout life, being modified – for better or worse – by the experiences of adulthood.

Much of what we know about well-being derives from the close study of mental ill health, because the latter is easier to grasp than the former. People who are able to respond effectively to the demands made upon them and are able to maintain roles that give them value possess a wellness that is specific to their circumstances and that gives them enormous flexibility. Those who cannot meet societal demands become distressed, anxious, depressed or develop psychotic symptoms and forms of behaviour that are near universal in their content. Mental wellness and mental ill health are always inseparable, being different ways of functioning in a given situation, and are not binary or mutually exclusive opposites but rather the ends of a spectrum of reactions to changing situations. The mentally well septuagenarian can enjoy sports, grandchildren and any form of recreation that is within their physical and financial limits but they can still be profoundly saddened by loss. The mentally ill septuagenarian can do less than they and others would want but rarely retreats into an uncommunicative or unresponsive state.

A socio-medical model of mental wellness and illness offers some hints about the complexity of the mechanisms that sustain or fail to protect well-being. Some things appear to be fundamental to vulnerability (causal factors), and some seem to prompt slippage into mental ill health in already vulnerable individuals (trigger factors). Policies and practices can be designed to minimize the impact of causal factors, so loss of mobility or worsening eyesight can be offset by changes to the built environment, to levels of illumination and to the presentation of the printed word, as well as in aids to physical activity or tools for enhancing vision. In England, recognition of the contributory factors of **social exclusion** in later life has gradually moved into the policy arena (see Box 4.1), though often reflecting physical and economic forms of exclusion rather than psychosocial ones. Our argument is that this kind of model applies to all forms of mental ill health. This is because mental well-being also has causal factors that are fundamental to well-being as well as reinforcing factors that sustain wellness.

---

### Box 4.1 *Sure Start to Later Life*

The Social Exclusion Unit (SEU 2006) report, *A Sure Start to Later Life: Ending Inequalities for Older People*, builds on the multidepartmental policy document *Opportunity Age* (DWP 2005) by recognizing that the aspirations of independence, dignity, choice, quality of life, and the inclusive communities that underpin these, cannot be realized for older people who experience social exclusion. It identifies a need to ensure basic standards of health and wealth and to address the housing needs of older people. The report highlights three contributory factors leading to social exclusion in later life:

- People who are excluded in mid-life are unlikely to be able to break the cycle of exclusion in later life; indeed it can often become more acute.
- Life events, such as bereavement, can lead people to become excluded in later life.
- Pervasive and cumulative age discrimination saps the aspirations of individuals and the environment within which they operate – leading to exclusion.

*Sure Start to Later Life* argues that these exclusions become compounded by the failure of services to react to the complexity of exclusion in later life.

---

A schematic example of this is shown in Figure 4.1, which is a hypothetical model of late life depression (McQuellon and Reifler 1987), which fits the available epidemiological and observational evidence and offers a range of opportunities for practice intervention. However, this model of causal and trigger (or reinforcing) factors is abstract and highly generalized so is difficult to apply to policy. It does not tell us why psychological resilience and vulnerability are so variably spread in the population, why causal factors affect some but not others and why triggers or reinforcers fail to work in many people while they function as the model predicts in other people. We need to understand why the majority of older people who experience adverse events or social exclusion do not become depressed, even if most depressed older people have had a recent adverse event that appears to have triggered their depression. There must be some factors that protect us, as we age, against the accumulative effects of a series of adversities and challenges. These factors are variously termed 'coping strategies', 'resilience' or 'self-efficacy', and all imply that individuals actively make sense of their situation as it changes, and as they encounter physical or psychosocial threats and risks. Although mental wellness and mental ill health are not 'all in the mind' – the former is a very social state in many ways, and the latter very physical – their significance and impact depend very much on how we think about them.

We can see how the ways in which we view mental wellness influence how we behave and therefore how policy and practice can affect well-being, by pursuing the example of depression in later life further. Older people with mental health problems often believe that the primary responsibility for combating their symptoms lies with themselves, with external support being a secondary consideration. Nevertheless, they also welcome opportunities to discuss their problems with professionals, particularly

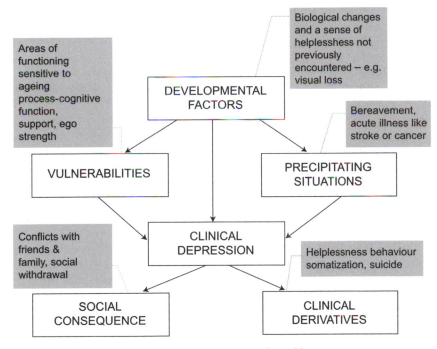

**Figure 4.1**  A hypothetical model of depression in later life
*Source*: Modified from McQuellon and Reifer (1987)

general practitioners (GPs) (Lawrence et al. 2006). This is not as contradictory as it sounds because discussion does not necessarily imply transfer of responsibility. Professionals may see themselves as 'active managers' and 'problem solvers', but those seeking their advice may want no more than advice. In the example of depression, older people may retain the sense of agency that is so central to their mental well-being.

GPs' perceptions of depression in older people to some extent match those of their patients, in that depression is seen as being a consequence of adverse personal and social circumstances. But they also see depressed older people as passive, with low expectations of help (Burroughs et al. 2006) and with a tendency to discuss physical rather than psychological problems (Murray et al. 2006). Older people with depressed mood often believe that depression is due to stress or heredity, that its symptoms fluctuate over time but follow a chronic course, and that they can control their depressed mood by using coping mechanisms, but only up to a point. Significantly, these illness explanations can be modified through contact with professionals (and their different perspectives on depression) but the older people tend to revert to the original explanation over time (Brown et al. 2001).

There are some important lessons for policy and practice here for the model of well-being/ill-being that the older person has, that may be more complex and more differentiated than that of the professional. A policy to screen for depression in older people in primary care, then, is unlikely to be very beneficial if it leads to a clash of perceptions and to practice that is incongruent with the personal experiences and beliefs of the individual concerned. The professional or service commissioner view that drop-in centres or lunch clubs, for example, might be the mechanism for restoring and sustaining mental well-being for an individual could be equally unfounded.

Once again, we argue that the principles apply outside depression (as a collection of symptoms) to the whole spectrum of mental wellness/illness. One interesting finding is that close personal relationships with professionals could be experienced as either supportive or as a barrier to communication when discussing psychological symptoms (Emslie et al. 2007). Therefore, a person with a very long and positive relationship with their GP or practice nurse may be reluctant to raise such concerns, and the professionals may wonder why the locum or agency nurse seems to have found something that they have missed. Another message for professionals working with older people whose mental well-being is impaired is that those who rate highly on self-help capabilities also rate highly on help-seeking from others (Zauszniewski 1996). A professional focus that aims to reduce help-seeking behaviour by increasing self-help behaviour may be missing the point; help-seeking creates the opportunities to enhance self-help, which appears to be an effective anti-depressant (Zauszniewski 1996). Such thinking resonates with policy goals that illustrate the importance of prevention in English social policy for older people (see Box 4.2).

---

**Box 4.2** White Paper for primary and community care

The White Paper for primary and community care: *Our Health, Our Care, Our Say: A New Direction for Community Services* (DH 2006) reinforces the emphasis on independence, choice and well-being, and aims to achieve four goals:

- better prevention services with earlier intervention;
- more choice and a louder voice for patients;
- more action to tackle inequalities and improve access to community services;
- more support for people with long-term needs.

---

### Does gender matter?

Other effects may compound the biographical complexities of mental wellness and illness. Everyone knows that 'men are from Mars and women from Venus', so it is common sense that men and women might experience mental wellness and illness differently. However, while there are many stereotypes about gendered responses to psychological distress, there is little firm empirical evidence to inform policy and practice. There are some grounds for thinking that gender differences in help-seeking are less apparent in older than in younger adults, especially among those seeking help for psychological problems (George 1990), but given the variety of biographical experiences between men and women, we might still need to understand even small differences. There may be some important lessons to be learned from the perceptions that younger adults have of mental wellness and illness. For example, there is some evidence that both men and women find it equally difficult to recognize and articulate mental health problems, with negative consequences for the ways in which they communicate with professionals (Emslie et al. 2007). Men tend to value professional skills that help them to talk while women value listening skills (Emslie et al. 2007). Men commonly draw on 'masculine' values of re-establishing control and being responsible for others, as ways of coping with disturbances of mental well-being and psychological distress (Emslie et al. 2006). Women, on the other hand, may moderate the risk of depression by seeking religious help (if only by individual prayer) or by discussion of the adverse circumstances with others (Wang and Patten 2002). Understanding older people's coping mechanisms and repertoires of learned skills – attributes of active problem-solving agents rather than of passive and undemanding sufferers – may be crucial to developing policies and practices that promote or restore mental well-being in later life, and in enhancing the skills of professionals.

### What promotes mental well-being in later life?

There appear to be several mechanisms that sustain mental well-being, or at least reduce the severity, chronicity or impact of mental ill health. The overlapping ideas of 'self-efficacy' and 'learned resourcefulness' provide some clues. Self-efficacy reflects a person's optimistic self-belief about being able to change (Bandura 1977). The higher a person's self-efficacy, the more likely they are to put effort into a task, and recover from setbacks in the process (Schwarzer 1992). Self-efficacy is associated significantly and negatively with pain-related disability, and the experience of depression and depressive symptoms (Turner et al. 2005). Self-help strategies (learned resourcefulness) are significantly associated with better adaptive functioning (Zauszniewski 1996). In policy terms, these may be framed as the promotion of independence and control (see Box 4.3).

---

**Box 4.3** *Opportunity Age*

*Opportunity Age* (DWP 2005) set out the government's strategy and supporting evidence for developing the nation's approach to managing the well-known demographic changes over the next few decades. *Opportunity Age* suggests the following priorities for action:

- to achieve higher employment rates and greater flexibility for people aged over 50 years, managing any health conditions and combining work with family (and other) commitments;
- to enable *all* older people to play a full and active role in society, with an adequate income and decent housing;
- to allow us all to keep independence and control over our lives as we grow older, even if we are constrained by the health problems that can occur in old age.

---

### What increases vulnerability to mental health problems?

The risk, severity, chronicity and impact of mental health problems in later life seem to be determined by a narrow range of learned responses to adversity. Personality characteristics like 'neuroticism' are associated with highly emotional coping responses in major depression (Uehara et al. 1999). Greater emotional reaction to depression is associated with maladaptive coping for both men and women. Women differ from men because those women who have adaptive coping techniques appear to have greater perceived control over depression and are less likely to be disabled by depressive symptoms (Kelly et al. 2007). The tendency to 'catastrophize' adversity (to respond to all losses and harms as disasters) predicts the development of depression symptoms (Turner et al. 2000). Older people with more depressive symptoms use a passive form of acceptance, rumination and catastrophizing to a significantly higher extent, rather than 'positive re-appraisal' – where adverse events are actively integrated into their perception of the situation and the person adapts accordingly (Kraaij et al. 2002). On the other hand, individuals who use coping strategies that include problem solving and social support seeking have fewer symptoms than those who use escapist and avoidant strategies (like wishful thinking) (Vollman et al. 2007; see also Chapters 2 and 3).

## Policy implications

The policy implications of these perspectives are clear; anything that enhances self-efficacy and learned resourcefulness should be promoted, particularly in early life when basic coping mechanisms are established. Efforts in promoting parenting styles that foster these attributes are long-term strategies (e.g., Sure Start, see: http://www.surestart.gov.uk/publicationsandresources). Organizing education around their promotion, and recognizing and responding to the erosion of mental wellness in the teenage years all appear rational. It is heartening that primary prevention (developing effective coping strategies) shows some evidence of success – (see SEU 2004) and the Partnership for Older People's Projects (POPPS) initiatives seem promising in the efforts of some these projects to focus on primary prevention over the long term (see DH 2007c).

Herman (2001) argues that promoting community understanding about mental health and mental illness is the key to changing polices, not just in health but also in education, employment and the law. Respect for human rights is another thread that can influence responses to mental health problems by addressing stigma (Thornicroft 2006). Stigma is one aspect of mental health problems that may be compounded for older people, particularly those from culturally diverse backgrounds (Rait et al. 1996). Thus community development initiatives that enable older people to help themselves and each other, such as those that promote peer support, may be as effective in promoting mental wellness as they are in supporting people with mental health problems (Age Concern 2007).

Mainstreaming mental health promotion means addressing social isolation as well as enhancing existing social networks. Social inclusion policies have exposed the complexity of this and the multiple risk factors of isolation and loneliness. They have revealed that older people are easily isolated as a group from public policy strategies unless specifically identified. The evaluation of the National Service Framework for Older People (Healthcare Commission 2006) addressed some of the interlocking features of communities that may affect social connectedness, whether this is the effect of limited public transport, or perceptions and experiences of crime and disorder, or social change that has by-passed older residents in their neighbourhoods.

For policy-makers, one key question is how to develop or sustain coping strategies among future generations of older people. Policy is often accused of being short term, but health is one area where increasingly there is interest in forecasting and future-proofing, with due acknowledgements of the limits of such approaches. Interventions may have a sound economic rationale, since good mental health in later lives benefits everyone; they maximize the contributions to society that older people can make and bring benefits to society by reducing the costs of poor mental health in later life (Age Concern 2006: 16–17).

In policy terms, this enables a greater focus of support for particular groups of older people whose resilience or coping may be compromised by limited investment in their well-being and the ill effects, damage and distress of poverty and social exclusion. Loss of or diminishing peer and social networks, especially in very late old age, is not an area of public policy that has traditionally received more than token efforts. The inclusion of a commitment to tackle social isolation and loneliness by a powerful combination of cross-government bodies (DH 2007b) may encourage greater attention beyond the 'usual suspects' of health and social care providers. As Phillipson and Scharf (2004) observe, government policy affects vulnerable older people in complex ways. Improvements appear to have been made in addressing age-related characteristics that put particular pressures on people in retirement, such as stabilizing or reducing the numbers in relative poverty. Similarly, measures designed to tackle age-based discrimination seem to be producing a cultural shift in public perceptions of older people, in the sense that ageism is seen to exist but it is no longer acceptable. Those of us with interests in older people's services may not always appreciate these wider shifts in public attitudes.

We know that reducing avoidable adversity *and* increasing internal capacity strengthens coping during later life. This is why a primary prevention policy approach will increase:

- education and access to opportunities;
- control over the timing, type and scope of work;
- secure employment;
- safety within the home and within relationships;
- good housing.

In England, integrated policy, as set out by *Opportunity Age* (DWP 2005, see Box 4.3) and the relaunched *Carers Strategy* (DH 2008), aims to promote older people's well-being and to prevent mental ill health. It is likely to be the success of these policies, among others, that make the difference to primary prevention of depression as much as any policy directly aimed at health care and treatment. *Putting People First* (DH 2007b) sums up this approach (see Box 4.4), with its emphasis on early intervention.

---

**Box 4.4** *Putting People First*: the personalization agenda

**Policy goals of personalization**

In the public services strand of the government's policy review, *Building on Progress: Public Services* (Cabinet Office 2007), the government's approach to personalization is summarized as 'the way in which services are tailored to the needs and preferences of citizens. The overall vision is that the state should empower citizens to shape their own lives and the services they receive'.

The transformation of social care signalled in the Department of Health's (DH) social care Green Paper, *Independence, Well-being and Choice* (DH 2005) and reinforced in *Our Health, Our Care, Our Say: A New Direction for Community Services* (*DH 2006*) was confirmed in the concordat *Putting People First* (DH 2007b).

The aim of personalization is to ensure that everyone who is eligible for social care support – regardless of their level of need; in any setting; whether from statutory services, the voluntary and community or private sector, or from public funds or by funding it themselves – has more choice and control over what that support is, how it is delivered and by whom. If effective, it will mean that people are better able to live their own lives as they wish, confident that available services are of high quality, are safe and promote their independence, well-being and dignity.

*Putting People First* (DH 2007b) set out several policy goals that are highly relevant to the lives of current and future older generations. These include:

- the development of personal budgets;
- a commitment that local authorities and the NHS will not use 'poor performers';
- the development of First Stop Shops – providing information, advice and advocacy, available to people paying for their own social care;
- tackling loneliness and isolation;
- promoting intergenerational activities;
- investment in new technologies;
- prevention of disability and early intervention to address problems; that may be helped by timely support.

## Secondary prevention: a public health perspective

Our argument is that mental ill health at a societal level can be understood by adopting a public health perspective that allows a complex picture of causality to be seen. In this perspective, mental health is seen as being *determined* by causal factors like acquired coping strategies, socio-economic status, gender and migration, and *modified* by sources of heterogeneity, like lifestyle, experiences of adulthood and of social relationships, over a life course (Hertzman et al. 1994). This can be expressed pictorially, as shown in Figure 4.2, and allows us to reconsider the factors that might influence the appearance of mental health problems, and both lay and professional responses to them. The factors on the vertical and horizontal axes of the matrix interact throughout life, changing the health status of the person and creating individuals who become increasingly different from each other, as they get older. The older population is heterogeneous in ways that the diverse population of children is not, because more interactions have accumulated over time. Genetic factors may only be expressed later in life, and sometimes only when other changes have occurred. For example, Huntingdon's disease appears in middle age, often after the reproductive phase of life, and type 2 diabetes is much more common in older populations than in the younger, especially when obesity also develops.

The complexity of this perspective offers us multiple routes into policy and practice that could potentially promote mental well-being in an ageing population. Some, such as socio-economic status, environmental characteristics and access to resources, are obvious. Reducing poverty among older people, ensuring a safe environment, and making health and social services accessible to them are tasks that national and local government understand, even if they sometimes fail to act on them as well as they might. Creating enticing environments – libraries full of computers, leisure centres friendly to older people, well-serviced allotments, broad-band made available to every home together with the training to use it, opportunities for learning, diverse possibilities for volunteering – are ways to promote pleasure, usefulness, and self-efficacy. The complexity of this epidemiological perspective also allows us to understand the variable responses and vulnerabilities of individuals to adversity, even if few can necessarily predict the susceptibility of any individual as they age.

Within this perspective, we can begin to describe possible models of mental health promotion and maintenance, at least at community level, in terms of:

- how interactions between gender and sexuality, ethnicity and belief system, and lived experiences of older people influence mental health in later life;
- the interrelationship between mental ill health and physical disabilities. For example, efforts to reduce the risk of heart disease and stroke by promoting exercise, healthy eating and smoking cessation are likely to have positive effects on mental well-being, by reducing disability;
- the role of social relationships (including work relationships) in shaping and supporting mental health and ill health;
- the impact of socio-economic status/deprivation, including housing and the environment;
- the effects of migration and ethnicity on mental health in later life.

It is beyond the scope of this chapter to describe all these different dimensions of mental health promotion but more detail is provided in the other chapters in this book.

# Tertiary interventions: maximizing wellness in individuals

The strongest of coping strategies can be overcome, as the losses of ageing multiply. Those who lose their social roles, members of their peer group, their good health and their abilities will find it increasingly difficult to meet the demands of their society and environments with their available physical and psychological resources, and can develop the disability we call mental ill health (Verbrugge and Jette 1994). Anxiety and depression are sometimes the consequence, and can be particularly disabling, especially in those who have experienced them, even intermittently, in earlier life, or if they accompany problems such as dementia.

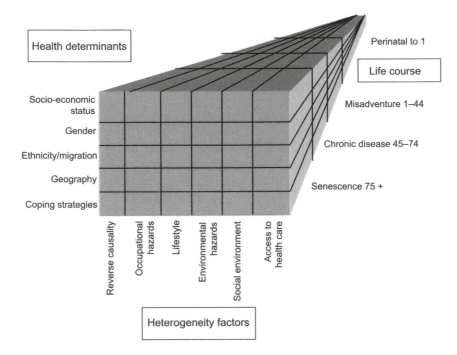

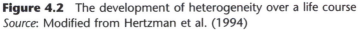

**Figure 4.2** The development of heterogeneity over a life course
*Source*: Modified from Hertzman et al. (1994)

Prevention of further harm and distress (through minimizing adverse events), of course, is linked to primary and secondary prevention since the effects of many adverse events in later life cannot be extinguished. Moreover, social exclusion arising from cumulative disadvantage appears more resistant to change (SEU 2004). Nevertheless, minimizing adverse events needs consideration and specific desirable public policy responses include:

- Enhanced support for carers (Age Concern 2007);
- Crime prevention and safeguarding (SEU 2004).

Both of these examples are designed, if implicitly rather than explicitly, to maximize coping strategies. While many coping strategies are forged early in childhood and teens, because all coping in later life stems from what is set early on, the strategies can become fragile and outside pressures may have enormous impact. The Age Concern / Mental Health Foundation Inquiry synthesis of prevention approaches in the literature (Age Concern 2006: 47) observed that support for carers could often be instrumental and allied to efforts to help younger carers return to work or to remain in employment, but that caring in later life was often under-recognized. Likewise, abuse and violence in later life, while not the totality of elder mistreatment and neglect, may contribute to depression and self-restricted social networks, when the fear of being taken advantage of or of younger people restricts social and community participation.

The relevance of policies associated with disability (for example, *Improving the Life Chances of Disabled People*, Strategy Unit 2005) is undervalued when thinking about secondary prevention of depression in policy terms. However, they highlight some of the policy goals and implementation strategies that might be useful to consider, particularly as a social model of responding to depression seems to hold out much promise (Manthorpe and Iliffe 2005). *Improving the Life Chances of Disabled People* sets targets for improving the life of disabled people. By 2025, for example, disabled people in Britain should have full opportunities and choices to improve their quality of life, and will be respected and included as equal members of society. It focuses on multi-government department issues and identifies barriers for disabled people that stall policies. Links to wide social inclusion agendas are explicit yet planning mechanisms are person-centred in relating agendas to individuals and removing the 'cliff faces of provision' (see Manthorpe and Iliffe 2008).

Tertiary prevention (treating and supporting older people with mental health problems) may seem less of a policy problem. If mental ill health in later life is more likely than not to be a chronic or long-term relapsing problem, then services need to remain engaged, and this is a matter for clinicians to organize. Nothing is that simple, however, and policy affects the nature of the workforce available; the capacity of teams to identify which patients need support, how and from whom; and whether older people are best serviced by legal and policy frameworks that focus on both choice and empowerment and on public protection and risk aversion. Many of these issues are more directly played out in relation to younger rather than older adults, but older people are still affected. *New Ways of Working* (DH 2007a), for example, may enable older people to benefit from teams that adopt a supportive multiskilled approach, since older people have often not had opportunities to access services such as counselling and therapy that are more often offered to younger adults. Older people, too will be affected by policies that aim to minimize the distress of 'revolving door' patients under the provisions of the Mental Health Act 2007 in England and Wales. In promoting greater empowerment and engagement with services, the provisions of the Mental Capacity Act 2005 may foster greater confidence among older people that their wishes will be taken into account. As we argued earlier, fostering this sense of agency seems to be emerging as an overarching theme in the subject of mental health promotion.

## Conclusions

It may be easier to promote protective coping strategies in children and young people than to repair less functional strategies in later life, and policies that have strengthened education and welfare may yet contradict the gloominess of those who doubt the robustness of younger generations. Nevertheless, policies and practices designed to maximize social inclusion, reinforce people's strengths and reduce adverse challenges – particularly those of work stresses, unemployment and poverty – are at the core of a population or community-level strategy against mental ill health in later life. Indeed they are the only realistic approach when best estimates are that there will be three million older people affected by mental health problems in later life in the UK by 2021 (Age Concern 2007). Individual responses, while necessary, may be more about limiting damage, containing distress and optimizing well-being. Much can be done to improve the quality of life of older people; there are no grounds for negative and nihilistic attitudes.

## Reflective questions

1   If you were asked to draw up an action plan to promote mental well-being among older people in your locality, what would be your first priority?
2   Thinking about older individuals whom you regularly encounter, what can you do individually to strengthen or improve their mental health?
3   What might be a way to encourage greater understanding of mental well-being in later life in your community?
4   How can we foster positive coping strategies for future generations of older people?
5   How can older people be involved in maintaining mental well-being for themselves and their peers?

## References

Age Concern (2006) *Promoting Mental Health and Well-Being in Later Life: A First Report from the UK Inquiry into Mental Health and Well-being in Later Life.* London: Age Concern/Mental Health Foundation.

Age Concern (2007) *Promoting Mental Health and Well-being in Later Life.* London: Age Concern/Mental Health Foundation.

Bandura, A. (1977) Self-efficacy: Toward a unifying theory of behavior change, *Psychological Review*, 84: 191–215.

Brown, C., Dunbar-Jacob, J., Palenchar, D. et al. (2001) Primary care patients' personal illness models for depression: a preliminary investigation, *Family Practice*, 18(3): 314–20.

Burroughs, H., Lovell, K., Morley, M. et al. (2006) 'Justifiable depression': how primary care professionals and patients view late-life depression. A qualitative study, *Family Practice*, 23(3): 369–77.

Cabinet Office (2007) *Building on Progress: Public Services.* London: Cabinet Office.

DH (Department of Health) (2005) *Independence, Well-being and Choice.* London: Department of Health.

DH (Department of Health) (2006) *Our Health, Our Care, Our Say: A New Direction for Community Services.* London: Department of Health.

DH (Department of Health) (2007a) *New Ways of Working.* London: Department of Health.

DH (Department of Health) (2007b) *Putting People First.* London: Department of Health.

DH (Department of Health) (2007c) *National Evaluation of POPP Projects: Interim Report on Progress.* Available at: http://www.dh.gov.uk/en/Publicationsandstatistics/Publications/PublicationsPolicyAndGuidance/DH_079422 (accessed 19 Aug. 2008).

DH (Department of Health) (2008) *Carers at the Heart of 21st Century Families and Communities: A Caring System on Your Side, a Life of Your Own*. London: Department of Health.

DWP (Department of Work and Pensions) (2005) *Opportunity Age*. London: Department of Work and Pension.

Emslie, C., Ridge, D., Ziebland, S. and Hunt, K. (2006) Men's accounts of depression: reconstructing or resisting hegemonic masculinity? *Social Science and Medicine*, 62(9): 2246–57.

Emslie, C., Ridge, D., Ziebland, S. and Hunt, K. (2007) Exploring men's and women's experiences of depression and engagement with health professionals: more similarities than differences? A qualitative interview study, *BMC Family Practice*, 8: 43.

George, L. (1990) Gender, age, psychiatric disorders, *Generations*, 14(30): 22–4.

Healthcare Commission (2006) *Living Well in Later Life*. London: Healthcare Commission.

Herman, H. (2001) The need for mental health promotion, *Australian and New Zealand Journal of Psychiatry*, 35(6): 709–15.

Hertzman, C., Frank, J. and Evans, R. G. (1994) Heterogeneities in health status and the determinants of population health, in R. G. Evans, M. L. Barer and T. R. Marmor (eds) *Why Are Some People Healthy and Others Not? The Determinants of Health of Populations*. New York: Aldine de Gruyter.

Kelly, M., Sereika, S., Battista, D. and Brown, C. (2007) The relationship between beliefs about depression and coping strategies: gender differences, *British Journal of Clinical Psychology*, 46: 315–32.

Kraaij, V., Pruymboom, E. and Garnefski, N. (2002) Cognitive coping and depressive symptoms in the elderly: a longitudinal study, *Aging & Mental Health*, 6(3): 275–81.

Lawrence, V., Banerjee, S., Bhugra, D. et al. (2006) Coping with depression in later life: a qualitative study of help-seeking in three ethnic groups, *Psychological Medicine*, 36(10): 1375–83.

Manthorpe, J. and Iliffe, S. (2005) *Depression in Later Life*. London: Jessica Kingsley.

Manthorpe, J. and Iliffe, S. (2008) The mental health of older people: taking a long view, *Journal of Integrated Care*, 16(4): 3–12.

McQuellon, R. P. and Reifler, B. (1987) Caring for the depressed elderly and their families, in G. A. Hughston, V. A. Christopherson and M. J. Bonjean (eds) *Aging & Family Therapy: Practitioner Perspectives on Golden Pond*. New York: Howarth.

Murray, J., Banerjee, S. and Byng, R. (2006) Primary care professionals' perceptions of depression in older people: a qualitative study, *Social Science and Medicine*, 63(5): 1363–73.

Phillipson, C. and Scharf, T. (2004) *The Impact of Government Policy on Social Exclusion Among Older People: A Review of the Literature for the Social Exclusion Unit in the Breaking the Cycle Series*. London: Office of the Deputy Prime Minister.

Rait, G., Burns, A. and Chew, C. (1996) Age, ethnicity and mental illness: a triple whammy, *British Medical Journal*, 313: 1347–8.

Schwarzer, R. (1992) Preface, in R. Schwarzer (ed.), *Self-efficacy: Thought Control of Action*. Washington, DC: Hemisphere Publishing Corporation.

SEU (Social Exclusion Unit) (2004) *Excluded Older People*. London: SEU. Available at: http://www.cabinetoffice.gov.uk/~/media/assets/www.cabinetoffice.gov.uk/ social_exclusion_task_force/publications_1997_to_2006/ excluded_older_responses%20pdf.ashx (accessed 19 Aug. 2008).

SEU (Social Exclusion Unit) (2006) *A Sure Start to Later Life: Ending Inequalities for Older People*. London: SEU. Available at: http://www.cabinetoffice.gov.uk/~/media/assets/ www.cabinetoffice.gov.uk/social_exclusion_task_force/publications_1997_to_2006/ a_sure_start%20pdf.ashx (accessed 19 Aug. 2008).

Strategy Unit (2005) *Improving the Life Chances of Disabled People*: *Final Report*. London: Prime Minister's Strategy Unit, Cabinet Office.

Thornicroft, G. (2006) *Actions Speak Louder: Tackling Discrimination Against People with Mental Illness*. London: Mental Health Foundation.

Turner, J., Ersek, M. and Kemp, C. (2005) Self-efficacy for managing pain is associated with disability, depression and pain coping among retirement community residents with chronic pain, *Journal of Pain*, 6(7): 471–9.

Turner, J., Jensen, M. and Romano, J. (2000) Do beliefs, coping and catastrophizing independently predict functioning in patients with chronic pain? *Pain*, 85(1–2): 115–25.

Uehara, T., Sakado, K., Sakado, M., Sato T. and Someya T. (1999) Relationship between stress coping and personality in patients with major depressive disorder, *Psychotherapy Psychosom*, 68(1): 26–30.

Verbrugge, L. M. and Jette, A. M. (1994) The disablement process, *Social Science & Medicine*, 38(1): 1–14.

Vollman, M., Lamontagne, L. and Hepworth, J. (2007) Coping and depressive symptoms in adults living with heart failure, *Journal of Cardiovascular Nursing*, 22(2): 125–30.

Wang, J. and Patten, S. (2002) The moderating effects of coping strategies on major depression in the general population, *Canadian Journal of Psychiatry*, 47(2): 167–73.

Zauszniewski, J. A. (1996) Self-help and help-seeking behaviour patterns in healthy elders, *Journal of Holistic Nursing*, 14(3): 223–36.

# 5   Work, retirement and money
## Suzanne Moffatt

## Editor's foreword

The previous chapters considered the wider aspects of mental health in relation to mental health promotion in later life. This chapter is the first chapter to take the issues to the level of older people's own perspectives of what matters and what impacts on their mental well-being. In the Scottish survey, which has been referred to earlier, older people highlighted that retirement and the transition into retirement could have a major impact on their mental health, both positively and negatively. The chapter starts with a brief historical overview of retirement and pensions, and some of the theoretical explanations of retirement and the experiences related to retirement. It provides empirical data on the health impact of retirement, and explores the factors involved in the decisions around retirement and how they impact on individuals' mental health. The chapter concludes by considering the hugely important issue of money and resources in later life, and how older people's mental health is affected by not having sufficient income to sustain themselves.

## Introduction

The period of retirement from work is longer now than at any previous time in history. In the UK, for example, men who reach state retirement age at 65 can expect a further 16.6 years of retirement and women of the same age can expect a further 19.4 years, if mortality rates remain the same as they were in 2003–05 (National Statistics 2006). Within economically developed countries, most people retire earlier than the state retirement age, further lengthening this period of post-working life (Ebbinghaus 2006). Adequate finances are key to avoiding poverty in retirement, and are themselves influenced by occupation, social class, gender, ethnicity and health status. Pension policies and wider economic conditions also have a bearing on income levels in later life. This chapter explores the connections between work, retirement and money and the ways in which each of these factors influence well-being in later life. The chapter begins with a very brief historical outline of retirement before giving an overview of the changing nature of retirement and pensions throughout the twentieth century. Next, a number of sociological perspectives on retirement are explored, followed by a more detailed consideration of experiences of retirement, early retirement, extending working life and the relationship between retirement and mental health in wealthy industrialized nations. Most of the literature on retirement, work and money relates to older people in economically prosperous countries. However, the topic of the following section draws attention to the majority of the world's older people who live in extreme poverty in the developing South. The remainder of the chapter focuses on the ways in which social class, gender and ethnicity influence the accrual of retirement resources and the profound influence that inadequate income has on the experience of retirement. Throughout the chapter, the reader is encouraged to think about the relationship between material resources and mental well-being and the wide-ranging impact of poverty in later life.

Mental health in later life is profoundly influenced by the complex web of factors that surround retirement, and these include: work, transition into retirement, financial security, health, retirement location, and family and friends. The next sections provide some historical and theoretical perspectives, and highlight the continually changing contexts within which retirement is shaped. Many of those currently retired are materially considerably better off than their parents were. This brief look at the history and theory of retirement indicates that future generations of retirees will have a diverse range of experiences, but perhaps within a climate of greater uncertainty. Successfully managing the risks and challenges of retirement is, arguably, essential to mental well-being in later life.

## Historical perspective on retirement

In the centuries preceding the introduction of widespread state retirement pension provision, various arrangements were made by older people in order to manage in their later years. The earliest available historical evidence dates back to the thirteenth century showing that retirement contracts were common in most peasant societies throughout Europe (Thane 2000). In return for care, shelter and/or an effective pension, the owner or tenant of property transferred their assets to another, usually although not always, a family member. The existing records relate to those with some means. Thane (2000) points out that the paucity of records about the poorest presents some difficulties in establishing how they managed, although,

> The poor of medieval and early modern England, and indeed in the nineteenth century and into the twentieth, struggled in an 'economy of makeshifts', that is, they patched together whatever resources they could gather in ever-shifting combinations: paid work when possible, growing food, use of common rights, help from family, friends, charity, poor relief, debt and begging. The struggle grew harder with advancing age and the components of the economy of each individual shifted gradually from dependence upon work to reliance on the help of others.

> (Thane 2000: 89)

This may seem to echo a distant era, but it is worth remembering that until well into the twentieth century, older people, particularly those in manual occupations did not retire. Retirement is therefore a relatively recent social phenomena within industrialized societies (Laczko and Phillipson 1991). Within less affluent countries, however, many older people live in extreme poverty, often with little or no means of financial support (HelpAge International 2006). This is compounded by changing patterns of family support in many countries, which have serious implications for economic security in later life (Aboderin 2004).

## Retirement and pensions

The German Chancellor Bismarck is credited with initiating the first state retirement pension scheme in 1889. This scheme provided for workers aged 70 and over at a time when average life expectancy was 45 years. Britain followed in 1908 with a meagre pension of five shillings for manual workers aged 70. At first, retirement was not noticeably affected by early pension provision because the age of qualification was so high compared to average life expectancy and the pension levels were low. Gradually, fewer workers remained in employment – in 1931 47.5 per cent of men aged 65 were recorded as such on the UK Census. The major shift resulted from the various welfare regimes emerging out of the industrialized nations after World War II. These systems were not uniform and Esping Andersen (1990) identified three main welfare typologies which have lead to markedly different levels of state pension provision (Middleton 2002); (see Box 5.1) .

---

**Box 5.1** Summary of main welfare state typologies

| Welfare state type | Characteristics | Example countries |
| --- | --- | --- |
| Liberal | Means testing, modest social insurance, strict entitlement rules, state encouragement of the market. | USA, Canada, Australia, UK. |
| Corporatist | Social insurance but preserves income differences. | France, Germany, Italy, Austria. |
| Social democratic | Redistributive. | Scandinavia: Sweden, Norway, Denmark. |

(Esping Andersen 1990)

---

Whatever the model adopted, state pension provision has been pivotal in consolidating retirement as an accepted social and economic institution throughout the industrialized nations which Phillipson (1998) regarded as the first phase in the modern history of retirement. However, compulsory retirement was not welcomed by all and there were several accounts of the difficulties experienced by some, mainly male manual workers, in adjusting to a work-free life (Townsend 1957), although as Thane (2000) points out, the fall in income and ensuing social and material loss would have been major influencing factors.

A second phase of retirement emerged from the mid-1980s onwards, characterized by the identification of a 'third age' between the period of work (the second age) and a period of physical and mental decline (the 'fourth' age) (Phillipson 1998: 84). Macro-level processes from the 1970s onwards brought about by the pressures of mass unemployment, contraction of traditional industries, schemes to promote redeployment and redundancies, and attitudes to older workers influenced working life in the later years as well as retirement transitions. Retirement is no longer a near universal experience marked by a fixed retirement age. Instead, this period is characterized by difference and diversity – there are now various pathways to retirement, such as unemployment, long-term sickness, redundancy or part-time employment.

> For the first generation of manual workers to experience retirement en masse in the 1940s and 50s, it was a sudden shock for which they were quite unprepared; for later generations it was an expected phase of life for which many more of them were better prepared, though it was still harder for many male manual workers than for better-off men and women for retired people of the 1960s and 70s it was an expectation for which they could plan

(Thane 2000: 403)

A number of economic, political and social factors have altered the experience of retirement from being a near universal mass experience to one which is now much more disparate and fragmented, and which defies any simple definition or categorization. Despite this, retirement is something that most people in industrialized countries now expect and experience.

## Sociological explanations of retirement

A number of sociological theories of retirement and later life have emerged, but the two most prominent concern: (1) the structured dependency of older people, and (2) the 'third age'. The theory of structured dependency is associated with British sociologists Townsend (1981), Walker (1981) and Vincent (1995) who argued that the low status and poverty widely experienced by older people were the unavoidable result of social policies which made retired people 'structurally dependent' on pensions or state welfare benefits. The widespread disadvantage resulting from the low level at which state pensions and benefits were set was not an inevitable aspect of later life. Furthermore, Townsend (2007) draws attention to ways in which the restriction of domestic and community roles artificially structures or worsens the dependency of older people. These ideas have been developed to emphasize structural factors affecting the lives of older women (Bernard et al. 1985; Ginn 2003) and ethnic minority elders (Evandrou 2000; Ginn and Arber 2000).

An alternative and more recent conceptualization of retirement emerges from the work of Peter Laslett (1989). Laslett characterizes retirement as a period relatively free from the obligations and pressures of paid work, and prior to the onset of serious health problems or disability. He argues that the simultaneous trends of increased longevity and earlier exit from the labour force enable a retirement period of enrichment and self-fulfilment. This theoretical position is concerned with the potential of a later life period which is no longer characterized by ill health and poverty. In the UK, this view has been most fully expounded by Gilleard and Higgs (2000, 2005) who show how increasing numbers of older people experience retirement as a period free from the constraints of work and a time for leisure, enjoyment and self-fulfilment. They argue that the trappings of 'old age' no longer dominate retirement and that this 'cultural turn' is embedded within wealthy industrialized societies, and is reflected in the many goods and services targeted at an older, affluent, non-working population (Gilleard and Higgs 2000, 2005). This perspective is the one most closely associated with positive mental health and well-being in later life.

Both positions can be said to represent extremes of the spectrum in industrialized societies, the former relating to the experiences of a substantial minority of older people who, as we shall see, still experience significant poverty, the latter describing the position of increasing numbers of older people with the resources and health to enjoy a fulfilling period of post-working life, and which represents the 'ideal' type of retirement in which individuals are free to choose to engage in activities and enjoy the company of family and friends.

## Experiencing retirement

There is a large body of international literature concerned with the consequences of retirement, drawing on a range of disciplines to assess the question: Is retirement good or bad for people? Its relevance is obviously in what it can tell us about retirement and positive mental well-being, with a view to creating policies which maximize the likelihood of retirement being a positive period for individuals. However, this research stems from a range of disciplines, with different theoretical underpinnings and methods and is of variable quality. Not surprisingly, much of the research evidence is contradictory and often difficult to generalize to populations other than those studied.

Studies of retired workers in the 1950s and 1960s have indicated that, for many, the transition into retirement was traumatic, and the period of retirement was one in which retired workers felt as though they were on the scrapheap, disengaged from society and reliant on inadequate incomes. The negative status of retirement persisted and perhaps even intensified in the 1980s as a result of the many forced redundancies of older workers from traditional industries in their late 50s and early 60s, who were treated as if they were retired. Higgs et al. (2003: 762) point out that retirement was seen as a marker of decline in social position, income and health. Other developments, driven particularly by the experiences of older white-collar workers with occupational and private pensions being offered attractive financial inducements to retire early, were leading to an increasing number of people entering a positive and fulfilling period of post-working life.

## Retirement and mental health

There has been a fairly widely held view that retirement is an event which can trigger ill health, with both physical and psychological problems (Minkler 1981), but there are now a number of studies which suggest that the transition into retirement may not in itself cause damage to an individual's health or well-being (Midanik et al. 1995; Fonseca and Paul 2004; Jaeger and Holm 2004). Rather, it is the particular circumstances which lead to retirement and in which retirement is experienced that influence mental health. Macro-social phenomena such as pension systems, societal norms regarding retirement are relevant here, as well as micro-social factors, for example, whether retirement is entered into voluntarily; physical and mental health, individual financial circumstances, family relationships and social networks; and how these factors interact with social class, gender, ethnicity and place.

Studies of depression in later life show considerable variation in prevalence across countries (Beekman et al. 1999) and within the UK (McDougall et al. 2007), but there appears to be fairly consistent evidence of higher levels of depression among women, older people with functionally limiting health conditions and those living in poor economic circumstances. Blane et al. (2008) found, using data from the English Longitudinal Study of Ageing (ELSA), that depression is likely to be an important factor affecting the beneficial and enjoyable aspects of ageing and that depression may play an important role in the functional limitations arising from various health conditions. There is also evidence that health and social inequalities increase in early old age (Chandola et al. 2007), and that such disadvantage is cumulative over the life course. Such evidence points to a relationship between micro and macro factors in later life which influences mental well-being. If poverty is a cause (albeit not the only one) of mental health problems in later life, one of the solutions is therefore to tackle poverty in later life.

Identifying the range of potential factors that influence well-being in later life is admittedly tricky, but one useful approach is that of the *life course*, a perspective which views retirement as one of several transitions throughout life that are embedded in historical, social and personal contexts which can be explored and therefore has considerable explanatory potential (Elder et al. 1996; Moen 1996). The following sections examine trends in retirement that can influence well-being and mental health.

## Recent trends in retirement

### Early retirement

Since the 1970s, early exit from the workforce has become increasingly widespread among the industrialized nations, and was once thought of as a solution to the

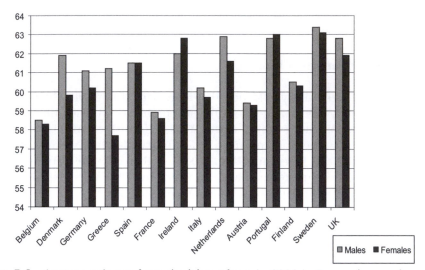

**Figure 5.1** Average exit age from the labour force in 2002 in Europe by gender
*Source*: International Labour Organization (2008)

problems of industrial restructuring and mass unemployment. The considerable cross-national differences in early retirement can be attributed to the particular welfare regime, pension system and economy of nation states. As Figure 5.1 shows, early exit from the workforce is widespread across Europe, although there is considerable variation between countries. Japan and the USA have lower levels of early retirement than Europe, although the trend has been in the same direction (Ebbinghaus 2006).

Research in the UK found that the most common reason for retiring (among half of the respondents) was ill health (Summerfield and Gill 2005). Other reasons for early retirement included wanting to enjoy life while still young and fit; having adequate income; and redundancy. The English Longitudinal Study on Ageing (ELSA) provides more detailed evidence about reasons for early retirement in the UK. Those aged over 50 not in work were disproportionately drawn from the poorest and the richest groups (Emmerson and Tetlow 2006). The richest were more likely to describe their exit from the labour market as retirement, in comparison to the poorest, who were more likely to withdraw because of ill health. This is borne out by another study which found that those who report poor health are more likely to move out of paid work and less likely to return to work (Solaiman Miah and Wilcox-Gok 2007). Ill health therefore has a significant effect on labour market participation for both men and women. Because of the known relationship between poor health, low pay and reliance on state benefits, the chances of building up sufficient resources for a comfortable retirement are slim among those on low incomes who retire early as a result of ill health.

To more fully understand the consequences of early retirement on well-being, we can draw on evidence from a small number of qualitative studies. Among a group of early retiring white-collar civil servants, those entering retirement with health problems were much less likely to perceive retirement as a period of opportunity: poor health constrained participation in post-retirement activities (Hyde et al. 2004). It was also found that those from the lower grades pursued fewer activities in retirement, and the authors suggest that this might have been because those from lower grades lacked the time or resources pre- and post-retirement to develop interests. Equally those from higher grades were more likely to have better access to public and private transport, and to live in areas with better facilities. Another study of white-collar civil servants found that decisions about early retirement were driven much more by economic factors than by physical health. However, stress loomed large, usually attributed to adverse work conditions, and Higgs et al. (2003: 771) suggest that, 'these results reflect a new pattern of early retirement in which mental health as well as economic considerations feature in the early retirement decisions among white-collar workers'.

Financial security and good health were key elements to leading a fulfilled post-working life – those who were better off in health and economic terms found it easier to participate. Barnes et al. (2002) found that adjustment to retirement was profoundly influenced by transition into retirement. Involuntary retirees, as a result of ill health, caring responsibilities or redundancy for example, had more problems adjusting to retirement, partly as a consequence of financial problems. Arthur (2002) found that a longer period of transition was beneficial because it allowed people more time to adjust psychologically and financially to retirement. These findings are backed up by an Australian study which showed that having control over the timing and manner of leaving work had a positive impact on psychological and social well-being in retirement (De Vaus et al. 2007). What really appears to matter to individuals is having control over when and how to retire. The evidence from British studies is that having a strong financial position and high occupational status leads to a high degree of choice and control over the transition to retirement, and that those with low to average earnings have restricted options (Arthur 2002). Another way of thinking about this is how an accumulation of factors over the life course such as income, wealth, employment conditions, health, social networks and relationships influence whether an individual has choice and control over how and when they leave the workforce.

## Working beyond the state pension age

Most OECD (Organisation for Economic Co-operation and Development) countries are actively pursuing policies to extend working life beyond existing state retirement. For example Germany has recently legislated for a universal extension to state pension age (SPA) from 65 to 67 years by 2012; current UK proposals indicate the intention to boost SPA to 68 years by 2044.

Cebulla et al. (2007) found that post-SPA employment rates in the UK were 8 per cent for both men and women, and likely to rise. There is very little empirical research among this group, but the available evidence shows that in addition to financial considerations, decisions are shaped by individual employees' marketable skills and the willingness of employers to accommodate older workers. Working longer may have consequences for domestic life, for example, the perpetuation of unequal domestic division of labour, and there is a need to examine such consequences further (Cebulla et al. 2007). Qualitative work by Parry and Taylor (2007) found that positive or negative feelings about working beyond state pension age depended on whether individuals had been able to make desired choices, and the congruence between a particular work orientation and specific financial, health and family circumstances.

The move to increase working time and postpone retirement might appear to be a sensible solution to increased life expectancy. However, social inequalities in life expectancy are found throughout all societies. For example, life expectancy in the UK varies dramatically depending on social class, gender and place. The 2001 UK Census data revealed that average life expectancy in Glasgow City was 69.3 years and 76.4 years, for men and women respectively, the equivalent figures for Kensington and Chelsea were 80.8 and 85.8 years respectively (ONS 2001). The drive to extend working life may exacerbate health problems among the least well, who are also those likely to be the poorest in society. While the move to extend working life may suit some individuals, it will not suit all, particularly those in poor health.

# Experiences of older people in developing countries

The majority of the world's population aged over 60 live in the developed world. By 2050, two-thirds of the estimated 1.2 billion people aged over 60 worldwide will live in developing countries, yet the overwhelming majority face an old age marked by serious financial insecurity and chronic poverty. Within low and middle income countries there are various models of pension provision, but only a small minority of older people are covered by contributory schemes, leaving the majority to rely on whatever state provision exists (Lloyd-Sherlock 2002). Social pensions provided to older people throughout the developing world are seen as a desirable solution to reducing poverty among older people and to have a positive impact on the household, acting to reduce child poverty, increase school enrolment and nutritional intake, as well as supporting overall economic growth. Moreover social pensions generally redistribute proportionately more income to women and therefore redress to some extent, the disadvantages faced by older women and, in some cultures, the severe discrimination faced by widows. Botswana, Lesotho and Nepal, among the poorest countries in the world, have domestically financed social pensions and HelpAge International (2006) is campaigning for universal social age pensions to start at 60 (see Box 5.2).

**Box 5.2** The impact of social pensions on older people in developing countries

The following examples from HelpAge International (2006) illustrate the usefulness of social pensions:

Dona Elvira, a Bolivian widow, uses the Bonosol (Bolivia's social pension) as capital to buy goods and then, with her relatives, resells the goods at a profit to meet basic household expenses.

Haatantala, a Zambian widower, qualified for a government scheme that provides him with US$6 per month. He has used this money to buy seed and hire local labour to plough and cultivate his maize field. He has chosen to grow his own food rather than immediately buy food to ensure that he will not have to beg from his neighbours.

Reflect on the following:

- What is the potential impact of small social pensions on older people and their families in the developing world?
- Consider the consequences for older people who do not receive such support in later life.

The vast majority of older people in developing countries continue to live with children or other family members. However, Aboderin (2004: S135) has demonstrated how a 'complex interplay between resource constraints and changing normative ideas' is leading to a decline in material support that signifies a break from past traditions among older and younger generations in Ghana. Urbanization, migration and increased female participation in the labour force produces constraints that resonate throughout communities in the developing world; some researchers argue that living arrangements in many developing countries are likely to shift more towards a Western pattern in subsequent decades. Moreover, it is misleading to equate co-residence with adequate informal care from family members.

It is sobering to consider how many of the world's older population do not have access to adequate income for basic needs, access to health care or social protection in later life. Most older people continue to make a substantial contribution by continuing to work in the informal sector through domestic labour and caring; in countries affected by AIDS/HIV, it is older people who are raising the next generation.

Adequate levels of social protection for older people in developing countries require serious policy reform as well as redistribution of resources from North to South.

**Money**

The transition into retirement corresponds with a drop in income. A key issue is whether this transition is associated with a greater probability of becoming poor

(Bardasi et al. 2002). We have seen that depression in later life is associated with social deprivation; conversely there is a strong relationship between wealth and life satisfaction: the wealthier people are in their 50s, 60s and mid-70s, the higher their levels of life satisfaction (Demakakos et al. 2006). This is not to suggest that money is the only cause of well-being in later life, but financial security is regarded by older people themselves as a key factor for a satisfactory retirement (Bostock and Millar 2003; Bowling and Gabriel 2007). The accumulation of resources over a lifetime is socially patterned and largely dependent on educational attainment and occupation, themselves influenced by social class, gender and ethnicity. Among industrialized countries with state pension provision, there are varying degrees of shift towards making individuals, rather than the state, responsible for income replacement after retirement. This has led to greater reliance on private sector pension provision. Although individuals in most industrialized countries are encouraged to develop appropriate retirement income through pension funds and other assets, considerable risks are attached which are borne by the individual. The extent to which state pension provision compensates for individual differences in lifetime resource accumulation varies throughout the industrialized world, and income inequalities are greatest in the highly privatized systems of the UK and the USA (Ginn 2004). Being in receipt of an occupational pension is not, in itself, a safeguard against low income in later life as many occupational schemes have yielded quite modest pensions (Ginn 2003), and uncertainties abound over the actual level of income which will be derived from occupational pensions (Gilleard and Higgs 2005).

## Socio-economic position

The ability to accrue assets for retirement is predominantly influenced by occupation. Occupations of higher socio-economic status are generally associated with higher salaries and benefits such as occupational pension schemes. Occupations at the lower end of the scale come with less financial reward, few benefits and greater levels of insecurity. Within Europe, Britain has the widest inequalities in income and this is reflected in the source and level of retirement income such that, by 2001 two-thirds of the income of the richest 20 per cent of retirees was derived from private sources in the form of occupational pensions, personal pensions, investments and property income (Gilleard and Higgs 2005). In stark contrast, the poorest UK pensioners are reliant upon the state for 90 per cent of their income (Victor 2005). The UK state pension is the lowest in Europe. While UK pensioners can apply for means tested benefits to increase their income to the EU-defined poverty rate of 60 per cent of the median income, a considerable proportion of these benefits are not claimed (Mayhew 2002; Moffatt and Scambler 2008). Non-take-up of state benefits is the greatest cause of pensioner poverty in the UK and disproportionately affects the poorest pensioners (Harrop and Palmer 2002).

## Gender

In spite of gender equality legislation, gender differences in occupational status, opportunities and hourly pay persist in the EU and other industrialized countries. The occupational position of women, coupled with the care commitments as a result of motherhood or caring for older family members, limits women's ability to contribute to pension schemes in most countries. As Ginn (2004) points out, most women are severely disadvantaged by pension systems in which maximum entitlements are acquired as a result of continuous full-time employment between the ages of 20 and 65. Ginn (2004) demonstrates that most European state pension systems have some provision to compensate for the interrupted pattern of women's labour force partici-pation, but notes that Britain stands out as having particularly low levels of state pension compared to other similar systems. Women are also less likely to be members of defined benefit occupational pension schemes which have the advantage of an employer contribution. Notwithstanding different welfare models (see Box 5.1), Ginn (2004) argues that state pension provision is better equipped than private provision to reduce the adverse effects of caring responsibilities, an interrupted career trajectory and lower pay. Current policies to reduce state pension benefits and encourage workers to rely on the private sector are likely to lead to an increase in pensioner poverty, particularly for women, manual workers and ethnic minorities, as well as increase inequalities in later life (Evandrou and Falkingham 2005).

## Ethnicity

Various post–war patterns of migration have led to substantial ethnic minority populations in most industrialized countries. Generally speaking, within industrial-ized countries, the age structure of ethnic minority populations is younger than that of the white majority, although the proportion of ethnic minority elders is increasing and will continue to do so. In the USA in 2006, minority elders made up 16.1 per cent of the total population aged 65 and older and this is projected to rise to 25 per cent by 2025. In the UK, the projected ethnic minority population over the age of 65 by 2030 is 1.7 million (Patel 1999). Ethnic minority groups are hugely diverse, however, and in all wealthy industrialized countries minority elders are over-represented in the lower income groups. Patterns of migration, interrupted work histories, unemploy-ment and low paid work negatively influence the development of adequate pension contributions, which in many cases leads to dependency on other family members. Although many minority elders expect care in their later years by younger family members, this is not always possible (Atkin and Rollings 1996).

Interestingly, work which has examined quality of life of older people from ethnic minority groups in the UK shows how some disadvantaged groups do particularly well in terms of social and community networks, and that despite the majority living in disadvantaged neighbourhoods, most perceive the quality of their neighbourhood as good (Bajekal et al. 2004). This reflects the benefits of strong local social and community networks brought about by patterns of residence which facilitate the building of community resources such as shops, places of worship and businesses (Grewal et al. 2004), and is: something that many seem to be able to draw on in their older ages in the context of ongoing significant economic hardship and poor health, has evidently done much to enhance the lives of at least some older ethnic minority people (Nazroo 2006: 71).

## Mental health and financial well-being

There is considerable evidence from surveys to show that women, ethnic minorities and the 'oldest old' are at greater risk of poverty and that inequalities in income in some industrialized countries are increasing among older people. We also know that the majority of older people in the developing world live in extreme poverty. Those who advocate social justice argue, rightly, that older people deserve to live their later years without the reality or fear of poverty. But what of the relationship between poverty and mental well-being in later life? Box 5.3 contains insights from older people in North-East England who received additional state welfare benefits that they did not know they were entitled to, and graphically illustrates the anxiety they experienced and the ways in which their opportunities to engage in social activities were severely curtailed as a result of low income.

---

**Box 5.3** Insights from older people living on a low income in North-East England

Mrs MacLeod and Mrs Parks qualified for state welfare benefits that they were unaware of. They reflect on what it was like managing on very low incomes and the impact of additional income.

Mrs MacLeod, aged 82, income increased by 51 per cent:

> I used to get so depressed that I couldn't afford this that and the other, and now you know, I think to myself, oooh look at my [bank] statement, I can afford that, that's lovely, it makes me feel good.

Mrs Parks, aged 82, income increased by 30 per cent:

> I was living on the bare pension [i.e., below the poverty line] it doesn't leave you much for entertainment, and I couldn't go very far, because that's why I stopped going to the [ex-service men and women's association], when they started to go away for weekends and different places for reunions and whatnot, well, I couldn't go because I couldn't afford to go. You see, now I could, it makes that difference. It's not a lot but just that little bit difference between not being able to afford anything above normal, to having a little bit of enjoyment and a little bit of entertainment.

Consider the following questions:

- What are the consequences of poverty in later life?

---

- How might inadequate material resources impact on mental health?

  (See Moffatt and Scambler (2008) for further examples)

Work in the UK that has facilitated access to previously unclaimed state benefits and increased older people's incomes to a still modest, but more adequate, level illustrates the constraints placed on older people's lives by inadequate resources (Moffatt 2008). Moreover, this work demonstrates the ways in which material resources underpin social relations and acceptable levels of participation in society. In essence, lack of adequate material resources in later life, whether in the developed or developing world, can and does have a direct and negative impact on mental well-being.

## Achieving well-being in retirement

Lack of money to engage in the norms and practices of a society influences well-being in retirement. However, there are features other than money which facilitate social participation and social integration among retirees. Transport, housing, public amenities and leisure facilities are crucial to facilitating engagement with what Gilleard and Higgs (2005) refer to as 'Third Age Culture'. Deprived neighbourhoods have disproportionately fewer facilities, further disadvantaging poorer older people from participating. Remaining socially engaged, an important aspect of well-being in retirement, is closely linked to mental well-being (Moen et al. 2000). However, the ability to remain socially engaged is strongly socially patterned, and influenced by the places in which older people reside (Scharf et al. 2005). Just as some people may be better equipped (financially, socially, educationally) to remain socially engaged, so too are some places more conducive to enabling older people to participate by means of decent transport, safe streets and accessible amenities.

Recognizing the importance of adequate finance to well-being in later life, many UK organizations campaigning on behalf of older people provide information designed to assist older people to maximize their incomes. Nationally, both Help the Aged and Age Concern provide comprehensive advice about claiming benefit entitlements, both websites stating that 'over £4.2 billion in means tested benefits goes unclaimed per year'. There are several reasons for non-claiming of benefit entitlements, but perhaps the most common are lack of knowledge and complexity of the system (Moffatt and Higgs 2007). There is no statutory scheme in place throughout the UK to provide older people with benefit advice. The existing advice provision, often of high quality, is largely poorly funded, short-term and geographically patchy. However, evidence shows that benefit campaigns specifically targeted at older people can be highly effective (CAB 2003). Considerable amounts of unclaimed benefits are recouped and this has a positive effect on well-being (see Box 5.3).

Evidence would also suggest that many older people find health settings particularly acceptable for accessing this type of advice, but there are also many practical reasons why linking welfare rights advice and health settings can be advantageous to older people and service providers: many older people, including the housebound, are in regular contact and are well known to health care providers as a result of receiving preventative services, or because of ill health, disability or their caring roles (Moffatt and Scambler 2008). Primary care is therefore a worthwhile setting in which welfare rights advice can be provided and is an area where health professionals should be more proactive. Ideally, health professionals should facilitate contact between older people and welfare rights specialists to ensure that older people are claiming what they are entitled to. Universal access to such services, which involves partnership between health trusts and a range of advice agencies would make a considerable contribution to improving older people's material well-being and mental health.

## Conclusions

The main argument of this chapter is that material adequacy is an essential element of well-being in retirement. Throughout the industrialized world, increasing numbers of older people are materially secure, but this is strongly influenced by social class, gender, ethnicity, occupation and disability. Ensuring adequate resources is now, more than ever, an individual responsibility (Hirsch 2003), and those who have not earned an adequate income throughout most of their working lives are severely disadvantaged. Within the developed world, substantial numbers of older people exist in material circumstances that exclude them from what the rest of society regards as an acceptable standard of living. Most older people in developing countries struggle to survive, yet the evidence shows that making social pension provision widespread is possible and would significantly reduce the severe hardships faced by millions of older people and their families.

The transition into retirement occurs across a wide age range, it may be entered into voluntarily or involuntarily, some people wish to extend their working lives, others do not. What is clear is that retiring is a major life transition and inevitably requires some adjustments. Acquiring a new sense of identity and purpose comes easier to some than to others, and remaining socially integrated is a key factor for well-being in later life.

This chapter has highlighted the close links between the material and the social. Inadequate income in retirement has a major influence on anxiety, stress and depression, and is a contributory factor to social isolation. Lack of adequate income is an infringement of fundamental human rights and denies older people everywhere their basic citizenship rights.

## Acknowledgements

I would like to thank Paul Higgs for his comments on an earlier draft of this chapter.

## Reflective questions

1   What factors over the life course accumulate to influence the degree of choice and control individual's have over how and when to retire?

2    Consider the impact of policies to extend working life. What differential effects might these policies have?

3    What policies might reduce later life inequalities in income?

4    What steps can professionals working with older people in the UK take to ensure that maximum benefit entitlement is being claimed?

## Suggestions for further reading

### Social welfare systems

Esping Andersen, G. (1996) *Welfare States in Transition: National Adaptations in Global Economies*. London: Sage.

Esping Andersen, G. (2002) *Why We Need a New Welfare State*. Oxford: Oxford University Press.

### Work, retirement and pensions

Evandrou, M. and Falkingham, J. (2006) Will the baby-boomers be better off than their parents in retirement? in J. Vincent, C. Phillipson and M. Downs (eds), *The Futures of Old Age*. London: Sage Publications.

Marshall, V. W. and Taylor, P. (2005) Restructuring the lifecourse: work and retirement, in M. L. Johnson (ed.), *The Cambridge Handbook of Age and Ageing*. Cambridge: Cambridge University Press.

Price, D. and Ginn, J. (2006) The future of inequalities in retirement income, in J. Vincent, C. Phillipson and M. Downs (eds), *The Futures of Old Age*. London: Sage Publications.

### Ageing and social protection in developing countries

Aboderin, I. (2004) Modernisation and ageing theory revisited: current explanations of recent developing world and historical Western shifts in material family support for older people, *Ageing and Society*, 24: 29–50.

HelpAge International: http://www.helpage.org/Home

Lloyd-Sherlock, P. (2002) Formal social protection for older people in developing countries: three different approaches, *Journal of Social Policy*, 31(4): 695–713.

Lloyd-Sherlock, P. (ed.) (2004) *Living Longer: Ageing, Development and Social Protection*. London: Zed Books.

## References

Aboderin, I. (2004) Decline in material family support for older people in urban Ghana: understanding processes and causes of change, *Journal of Gerontology: Social Sciences*, 59B: S128–S137.

Arthur, S. (2002) *Money, Choice and Control: The Financial Circumstances of Early Retirement*. Bristol: Policy Press.

Atkin, K. and Rollings, J. (1996) Looking after their own? Family care-giving among Asian and Afro-Caribbean communities, in W. I. U. Ahmad and K. Atkin (eds), *'Race' and Community Care*. Buckingham: Open University Press.

Bajekal, M., Blane, D., Grewal, I., Karlsen, S. and Nazroo, J. (2004) Ethnic differences in influences on quality of life at older ages: a quantitative analysis, *Ageing and Society*, 24: 709–28.

Bardasi, E., Jenkins, S. and Rigg, J. (2002) Retirement and the income of older people: a British perspective, *Ageing and Society*, 22: 131–59.

Barnes, H., Parry, J. and Lakey, J. (2002) *Forging a New Future: The Experiences and Expectations of People Leaving Paid Work over 50*. Bristol: Policy Press.

Beekman, A. T. F., Copeland, J. R. M. and Prince, M. J. (1999) Review of community depression in later life, *British Journal of Psychiatry*, 174: 307–11.

Bernard, M., Itzin, C., Phillipson, C. and Skucha, J. (1985) Gendered work, gendered retirement, in S. Arber and J. Ginn (eds) *Connecting Gender and Ageing: A Sociological Approach*. Milton Keynes: Open University Press.

Blane, D., Netuveli, G. and Montgomery, S. M. (2008) Quality of life, health and physiological status and change at older ages, *Social Science and Medicine*, 66: 1579–87.

Bostock, Y. and Millar, C. (2003) *Older People's Perceptions of the Factors that Affect Mental Well-being in Later Life*. Edinburgh: NHS, Scotland.

Bowling, A. and Gabriel, Z. (2007) Lay theories of quality of life in old age, *Ageing and Society*, 27: 827–48.

CAB (Citizens Advice Bureau) 2003 *Serious Benefits: The Success of CAB Benefit Campaigns*. Available at: http://www.citizensadvice.org/pdf_serious_benefits.pdf (accessed Jun. 2007).

Cebulla, A., Butt, S. and Lyon, N. (2007) Working beyond the state pension age in the United Kingdom: the role of working time flexibility and the effects on the home, *Ageing and Society*, 27: 849–67.

Chandola, T., Ferrie, J., Sacker, A. and Marmot, M. (2007) Social inequalities in self reported health in early old age: follow-up of prospective cohort study, *BMJ Online First*, doi:10.1136/bmj.39167.439792.55, 27 Apr.

Demakakos, P., Nunn, S. and Nazroo, J. (2006) Loneliness, relative deprivation and life satisfaction, in J. Banks, E. Breeze, C. Lessof and J. Nazroo (eds) *Retirement, Health and Relationships of the Older Population in England: The 2004 English Longitudinal Study of Ageing*. London: Institute for Fiscal Studies.

De Vaus, D., Wells, Y., Kendig, H. and Quine, S. (2007) Does gradual retirement have better outcomes than abrupt retirement? Results from an Australian panel study, *Ageing and Society*, 27: 667–82.

Ebbinghaus, B. (2006) *Reforming Early Retirement in Europe, Japan and the USA*. Oxford: Oxford University Press.

Elder, G. H. J., George, L. K. and Shanahan, M. J. (1996) Psychosocial stress over the life course, in H. B. Kaplan (ed.), *Psychosocial Stress: Perspectives on Structure, Theory, Life Course and Methods*. Orlando, FL: Academic Press.

Emmerson, C. and Tetlow, G. (2006) Labour market transitions, in J. Banks, E. Breeze, C. Lessof and J. Nazroo (eds), *Retirement, Health and Relationships of the Older Population in England: The 2004 English Longitudinal Study of Ageing*. London: Institute for Fiscal Studies.

Esping Andersen, G. (1990) *The Three Worlds of Welfare Capitalism*. Cambridge: Polity Press.

Evandrou, M. (2000) Social inequalities in later life: the socio-economic position of older people from ethnic minority groups in Britain, *Population Trends*, 101: 11–18.

Evandrou, M. and Falkingham, J. (2005) A secure retirement for all? Older people and New Labour, in J. Hills and K. Stewart (eds) *A More Equal Society? New Labour, Poverty, Inequality and Exclusion*. Bristol: Policy Press.

Fonseca, A. M. and Paul, C. (2004) Health and aging: does retirement transition make any difference? *Reviews in Clinical Gerontology*, 13: 257–60.

Gilleard, C. and Higgs, P. (2000) *Cultures of Ageing: Self, Citizen and the Body*. London: Prentice Hall.

Gilleard, C. and Higgs, P. (2005) *Contexts of Ageing: Class, Cohort and Community*. Cambridge: Polity Press.

Ginn, J. (2003) *Gender, Pensions and the Lifecourse: How Pensions Need to Adapt to Changing Family Forms*. Bristol: Policy Press.

Ginn, J. (2004) European pension privatisation: taking account of gender, *Social Policy and Society*, 3: 123–34.

Ginn, J. and Arber, S. (2000) Ethnic inequality in later life: variation in financial circumstances by gender and ethnic group, *Education and Ageing*, 15: 65–83.

Grewal, I., Nazroo, M., Blane, D. and Lewis, J. (2004) Influences on quality of life: a qualitative investigation of ethnic differences among older people in England, *Journal of Ethnic and Migration Studies*, 30: 737–61.

Harrop, A. and Palmer, G. (2002) *Indicators of Poverty and Social Exclusion in Rural England*. Cambridge: The Countryside Agency, CAX117.

HelpAge International (2006) *Why Social Pensions Are Needed Now*. London: HelpAge International.

Higgs, P., Mein, G., Ferrie, J., Hyde, M. and Nazroo, J. (2003) Pathways to early retirement: structure and agency in decision making among British civil servants, *Ageing and Society*, 23: 761–78.

Hirsch, D. (2003) *Crossroads After 50: Improving Choices in Work and Retirement*. York: Joseph Rowntree Foundation.

Hyde, M., Ferrie, J., Higgs, P., Mein, G. and Nazroo, J. (2004) The effects of pre-retirement factors and retirement route on circumstances in retirement: findings from the Whitehall II study, *Ageing and Society*, 24: 279–96.

Jaeger, M. M. and Holm, A. (2004) *How Stressful is Retirement? New Evidence from a Longitudinal, Fixed-effects Analysis*. Copenhagen: Centre for Applied Micreconomics, University of Copenhagen.

Laczko, F. and Phillipson, C. (1991) *Changing Work and Retirement: Social Policy and the Older Worker*. Buckingham: Open University Press.

Laslett, P. (1989) *A Fresh Map of Life*. London: Weidenfield and Nicholson.

Lloyd-Sherlock, P. (2002) Formal social protection for older people in developing countries: three different approaches, *Journal of Social Policy*, 31: 695–713.

Mayhew, V. (2002) Barriers to take up among older people – a summary of the research, in A. Fleiss (ed.), *Social Research Yearbook 2000/2001*. London: Department for Work and Pensions.

McDougall, F. A., Kvall, K., Mathews, F. E. et al. (2007) Prevalence of depression in older people in England and Wales: the MRC CFA Study, *Psychological Medicine*, 37: 1787–95.

Midanik, L., Soghijian, K., Ransom, L. and Tekawa, I. (1995) The effect of retirement on mental health and health behaviours: The Kaiser Permanent Retirement Study, *Journal of Gerontology: Social Science*, 50B: S59–S61.

Middleton, S. (2002) Transition into retirement, in H. Barnes, C. Heady, S. Middleton et al. (eds) *Poverty and Social Exclusion in Europe*. Cheltenham: Edward Elgar.

Minkler, M. (1981) Research on the health effects of retirement: an uncertain legacy, *Journal of Health and Social Behavior*, 22.

Moen, P. (1996) A life course perspective on retirement, gender and well-being, *Journal of Occupational Health Psychology*, 1: 131–44.

Moen, P., Fields, V., Quick, H. E. and Hofmeister, H. (2000) A life-course approach to retirement and social integration, in K. Pillemer, P. Moen, E. Wethington, and N. Glasgow (eds) *Social Integration in the Second Half of Life*. Baltimore, MD: Johns Hopkins University Press.

Moffatt, S. and Higgs, P. (2007) Charity or entitlement? Generational habitus and the welfare state among older people in North East England, *Social Policy and Administration*, 41(5): 449–64.

Moffatt, S. and Scambler, G. (2008) Can welfare-rights advice targeted at older people reduce social exclusion? *Ageing and Society*, 28: 875–99.

National Statistics (2006) Life expectancy at age 65 continues to rise. News release. London: National Statistics.

Nazroo, J. (2006) Ethnicity and old age, in J. A. Vincent, C. R. Phillipson and M. D. Downs (eds) *The Futures of Old Age*. London: Sage Publications.

ONS (Office for National Statistics) (2001) *Life Expectancy at Birth*. London: Health Variations Team, ONS.

Parry, J. and Taylor, R. F. (2007) Orientation, opportunity and autonomy: why people work after pension age in England, *Ageing and Society*, 27: 579–98.

Patel, N. (1999) *Ageing Matters – Ethnic Concerns*. Bradford: Policy Research Institute on Ageing and Ethnicity, University of Bradford.

Phillipson, C. (1998) Changing work and retirement: older workers, discrimination and the labour market, in M. Bernard and J. Phillips (eds), *The Social Policy of Old Age*. New Romney, Kent: Centre for Policy on Ageing.

Scharf, T., Phillipson, G. and Smith, A. E. (2005) Social exclusion of older people in deprived urban communities of England, *European Journal of Ageing*, 2: 76–87.

Solaiman Miah, M. and Wilcox-Gok, V. (2007) Do the sick retire early? Chronic illness, asset accumulation and early retirement, *Applied Economics*, 39: 1921–36.

Summerfield, C. and Gill, B. (eds) (2005) *Social Trends 3: National Statistics*. Basingstoke: Palgrave Macmillan.

Thane, P. (2000) *Old Age in English History*. Oxford: Oxford University Press.

Townsend, P. (1957) *The Family Life of Old People*. London: Routledge and Kegan Paul.

Townsend, P. (1981) The structured dependency of the elderly: a creation of social policy in the twentieth century, *Ageing and Society*, 1: 5–28.

Townsend, P. (2007) Using human rights to defeat ageism: dealing with policy-induced 'structured dependency', in M. Bernard and T. Scharf (eds) *Critical Perspectives on Ageing Societies*. Bristol: Policy Press.

Victor, C. (2005) *The Social Context of Ageing: A Textbook of Gerontology*. London: Routledge.

Vincent, J. (1995) *Inequality and Old Age*. London: UCL Press.

Walker, A. (1981) Towards a political economy of old age, *Ageing and Society*, 1: 73–94.

# 6 Relationships
## Denise Forte

## Editor's foreword

Relationships are immensely important among the personal resources that individual older people can draw on to adapt to and cope with the changes in life that are part of growing older. This chapter focuses on three types of relationships: social, intimate and intergenerational, (specifically that between grandparent and grandchild). After discussing the key concept of social networks and the complex issues of loneliness and isolation, the chapter goes on to examine how these relationships affect mental health and well-being. It considers the main factors and obstacles that older people face in maintaining their relationships and forming new ones. Several case studies illustrate some of the challenges older people face in different countries and cultures. Finally, the chapter discusses some strategies for promoting mental health and well-being.

## Introduction

This chapter aims to explore the meaning of relationships for older people and their role in promoting and maintaining mental health and well-being. Its focus is on the different types of relationships that older people experience and their impact on mental health and well-being in later life. Identifying what older people find helpful in relationships should help policy-makers and care service providers develop effective strategies to promote mental health and well-being in this age group.

Relationships are based on a complex set of interactions between two or more individuals, resulting in positive or negative outcomes for the individual's well-being. All relationships have a degree of interdependency in that people in a relationship provide emotional and/or instrumental support to each other. The quality of the support in the relationship varies, but when positive it provides a protective mechanism against mental health problems in later life. Social networks provide the framework within which relationships are formed and sustained, and thus social networking is very important for older people.

Older people experience a number of different relationships in their lives. Every new interaction an older person engages in has the potential for a relationship to develop. Three types of relationships are considered in this chapter: social (family and friends); intimate (heterosexual or homosexual); and intergenerational (specifically grandparenting). Psychologists have suggested that human beings have a basic drive to maintain caring interpersonal relationships. According to this view, people need both stable relationships and satisfying interactions with the people in those relationships. If either of these two ingredients is missing, people will begin to feel anxious, lonely, depressed and unhappy.

Definitions of well-being have been discussed in previous chapters and both the subjective and objective nature of the concept have been highlighted. This chapter builds on those definitions to examine the benefits older people gain through supportive relationships (Farquhar 1995; Wenger 1996, 2000) and the opportunities that such relationships provide for them to feel valued as important members of their networks and communities. Research has found that strong family and friendship networks rate highly in the list of factors older people rank as important in contributing to positive mental health and well-being (Bowling 1995; Bostock and Millar 2003; Victor et al. 2004; Wilhelmson 2005; Son et al. 2007; and Hutchison et al. 2008). Studies (Farquhar 1995; Bostock and Millar 2003) have found that, together with activities, social relationships and the quality of contact with others are the most important factors determining quality of life and well-being for older people.

However, not all relationships have a positive influence on well-being. Evidence from a number of studies, while supporting the value of relationships to a person's well-being, recognize that some relationships have a negative impact. This is especially true, for example, if the older person: is having a relationship with someone who is experiencing financial or mental health problems; is suffering bereavement or loss; is in a homosexual relationship which is not recognized or supported; and in some societies, feels their children are not fulfilling their duties according to their cultural expectations (Lloyd-Sherlock and Locke 2008; Yang and Victor 2008).

## Definitions and concepts

It is useful to outline some of the key concepts and theories that are relevant to a discussion of relationships and their importance to mental health and well-being. Research studies have focused extensively on the structure, functioning and supportiveness of human relationships – the social context in which people live and their integration within society. This is often termed 'social capital'. As well as examining the presence of healthy social networks, the concepts of loneliness and isolation are also important in the social world of older people. Indeed, 'loneliness is often used as an exemplar of social engagement, because it is a factor that is seen as being integral to quality of life in old age' (Gibson 2001: 107).

### Social networks

Much of the research on relationships to date has focused on the interactions of individuals with their social network, the size of that network and frequency of contact with it (Wenger 1992, 1994; Litwin 2001). One study (Fiori et al. 2008) identifies four clearly defined network types that specifically relate to well-being as follows (Fiori et al. 2008: 2004):

1 Diverse or diffuse.
2 Restricted or socially isolated.
3 Friend- and/or community-focused.
4 Family-focused.

These network types reflect existing models and theories of social relationships, such as the *theory of functional specificity* and the **convoy model of social relations**. In the functional specificity model, the importance of a wide social network (diverse or diffuse) is emphasized as here relationships appear to be linked to specific functions. In the convoy model, the emphasis is more on the quality rather than on the quantity of relationships. The importance of the diverse networks and their role in supporting well-being is reinforced by a number of other studies. For example, Wenger (1992) identifies five types of social networks that offer varying support to older people (Table 6.1).

Network types may shift in response to life events such as illness and deteriorating health or bereavement. However, these studies provide a framework for consideration of how older people see their networks supporting or failing to support their mental health and well-being. The diverse, diffuse or integrated network type that promotes high levels of social engagement is seen to provide the greatest well-being as it provides the older person with a greater number and range of people to draw on. Conversely, the restricted or socially isolated network types are associated with lower levels of well-being, where older people may be at greater risk of loneliness and social isolation (Fiori et al. 2008).

**Table 6.1** Social network types

| | |
|---|---|
| Local family dependent | Focused on nearby kin and with few peripheral friends. |
| Local integrated support networks | Involving close relationships with local friends, family and neighbours usually based on long-term residence and active involvement in the community and are associated with high levels of life satisfaction. |
| Local self-contained networks | Usually involve an arm's length relationship with at least one relative and are often associated with childless individuals or couples. Reliance is often on neighbours and networks are smaller and looser. |
| Wider community-focused | Active relationships with distant family but focus on local friends and neighbours and involvement in a number of different friendship groups. |
| Private restricted | Characterized by an absence of local kin and minimal contact with neighbours. A very small network typically of independent couples or dependent loners. |

*Source:* Adapted from Wenger (1992).

## Loneliness and isolation

Loneliness and social isolation are often used interchangeably in a vague and ill-defined manner to indicate how individuals evaluate their overall social network and levels of engagement (Cattan et al. 2005). Loneliness can be said to describe the state in which there is a gap between the individual's actual and desired level of social engagement and as such is inherently subjective. Loneliness needs to be distinguished from concepts such as 'being alone' (time spent alone) and 'living alone' (a description of household arrangements). Social isolation, on the other hand, refers to the level of integration of individuals and groups into their wider social environment (Victor et al. 2004).

There is a complex relationship between the three concepts of loneliness, social isolation and living alone. While loneliness is not directly linked to living alone, there is some evidence to suggest that older people living alone are at increased risk of loneliness and/or social isolation (Wenger 1996), and that their levels of social engagement and breadth of social network may be limited. It has also been suggested 'that a contributing factor to loneliness is the social stigma attached to being alone' (de Jong Gierveld 1989, in Cattan et al. 2003: 21).

Typically theories of loneliness focus upon the impact it has on an individual's quality of life and ability to function in society. Witzelben (1968) distinguishes existential loneliness from secondary loneliness, the former is something that is born in all of us while the latter results from the loss of someone or something that is important to us. Weiss (1973 in Victor et al. 2004) designates loneliness as emotional or social. Emotional loneliness occurs as a result of a lack of close intense personal relationships, whereas social loneliness occurs as a result of limited social networks and a lack of social engagement. Working with older people it is important to differentiate between emotional and social loneliness as they may require different interventions (Cattan et al. 2003).

*Older people's experience of loneliness*

In a sample of over 1000 older people 61 per cent rated themselves as never lonely, 31 per cent as sometimes and only 5 per cent as often lonely (Victor et al. 2004). Older people experience loneliness in different ways and for different reasons. In one study (Victor et al. 2004), participants felt that loneliness was not an isolated concept and could vary across the lifespan and from day to day. It could be either as a result of a sudden change in circumstances such as bereavement or it could be more insidious, arising from an accumulation of life circumstances. Although the intensity of loneliness may change, for many older people there remains an underlying awareness of loneliness. The following case study (Box 6.1) illustrates one older person's experience of emotional loneliness and its impact on her mental health and well-being.

---

**Box 6.1** Social networks and loneliness

The following case study highlights the differences between the subjective nature of loneliness, and the more objective nature of social isolation. It also suggests that quality of relationship rather than quantity promotes mental health and well-being.

Marjory is 92 years old and lives independently. She was widowed 18 years ago and has lived on her own ever since. For some years she had a male companion who accompanied her on outings and holidays. She felt that after her husband's death her friend also became her confidant. However, five years ago his health deteriorated. He moved to a care home and died shortly afterwards. Marjory felt guilty that she had not been able to prevent his admission to the care home and was adamant that she did not want to be admitted to a care home under any circumstances.

She has a large circle of friends from different aspects of her life and these continue to provide support and companionship. She is active in the University of 3rd Age, enjoys swimming, attending a lunch club and going to concerts. Friends continue to give support and provide transport to her various activities. Despite this, she frequently reports feeling great loneliness, 'as she has no family living in the United Kingdom'. Her son and daughter live in Australia, but it is her son who causes her feelings of loneliness and of being alone. She often complains that he has not rung for some weeks and that this makes her feel disappointed and low.

Both her son and one of her granddaughters keep in touch regularly by telephone but this does little to allay her feelings of being neglected and her perception that her son does not ring often enough. The regular nature of the phone calls is not enough to address her sense of loneliness. She worries that there will be no one around were she to die, because her son is so far away. He has visited recently but this has only heightened the sense of loss and loneliness.

Recently she has become unwell, and this has added to a loss of mental well-being and the early signs of depression. The only thing she really wants is for her son to live close by, and to provide the support she feels she may need as her illness progresses.

---

*Risk factors for loneliness*

Studies in the 1940s, 1950s and 1960s examined the nature and degree of social engagement among older people, to identify and measure the extent of loneliness and social isolation in later life, and to identify risk indicators for this population (Sheldon 1948; Townsend 1968). Victor et al. (2002) identified six factors which were likely to place an older person at greater risk of loneliness:

1   Poor health.
2   Increased time alone.
3   Mental health problems.
4   Being unmarried.
5   Increased perception of loneliness.
6   Health worse in old age than expected.

The Scottish mental health survey, previously referred to, identified five stages of vulnerability increasing older people's risk of loneliness and social isolation. They focused on key life events: 'pre-retirement; bereavement; selling the family home and moving into care' (Bostock and Millar 2003: 38). Any attempt at promoting well-being and mental health in older people needs to take account of their support needs at times of vulnerability.

Participants in one study (Victor et al. 2004) identified 27 factors that cause loneliness and these were grouped into four domains: family and friendship networks; community networks; activities and functional limitations; and personality factors (found to be of lesser importance). The same study found protective factors against loneliness in old age were advanced age and possession of educational qualifications. This was supported by findings from a Swedish ten-year follow-up study (Holmen and Fukurama 2002) where reported loneliness among people aged over 75 fell from 35.6 per cent in the initial study to 4.6 per cent at the third follow-up interview, suggesting that those that survived had learned to adapt to the vicissitudes of old age.

# Important attributes of relationships

Relationships are complex but the attributes considered most important for the mental well-being of older people include positive self-perception, reciprocity, and social and cognitive engagement.

## Self-perception

In the previously mentioned survey of older people, 'having a positive attitude was seen as contributing towards mental well-being. This was often linked to having a sense of values and to being open and tolerant of new ways of doing things and being willing to learn' (Bostock and Millar 2003: 5). All too often older people are seen as being resistant to change with limited potential for learning new ways of doing things. In other studies positive attitudes have also been found to be extremely beneficial in supporting older people to adapt to transitions and changes in later life (Keller-Cohen et al. 2006; Clemence 2006; Son et al. 2007; Hutchison et al. 2008). For some older people positive attitudes may be an inherent part of their psyche but for others they may be developed through the support they derive from their social networks (Keller-Cohen et al. 2006).

We experience our sense of self in relation to others; our individual identity is tied up closely with our social connections, as we sustain our own 'story' through others. Thus relationships are fundamental in reinforcing the individual's sense of identity and value. Growing older brings many challenges to this sense of identity and how individuals react will depend on the values and attitudes developed over a lifetime which enable them to adapt to change. Bowlby (1988) suggests the attachments formed in childhood and throughout the life cycle will have a major impact on the way individuals form attachments as they adjust to old age. Good interpersonal skills are also essential for supporting the individual's sense of self and self-identity. Edwards and Chapman suggest that 'interpersonal communication is central to the ageing process and provides some link between health and successful ageing being valued as a person implies being talked to and listened to' (2004: 16). These are essential components in establishing value and positive well-being in the older population and are reinforced by the relationships older people have in their lives, whether with family or friends, informal or formal carers, and with society as a whole.

## Reciprocity

Older age tends to be associated with increasing dependency on others which can undermine the normal balance of 'give and take' in relationships. Many studies cite the importance of reciprocity in relationships which enables older people to feel valued as equal partners in their interactions (Moriarty and Butt 2004; Keller-Cohen et al. 2006; ; Hutchison et al. 2008). Other studies have found benefits that accrue from reciprocal relationships include greater dignity, a sense of worth and greater satisfaction in accepting care from a family member if the older person has something to give back to the relationship (Wilson 1994; Son et al. 2007). These attributes all have a positive impact on well-being and mental health in later life. In an online survey of participation in the Red Hat Society, a women's leisure-based group operating in the USA and 30 other countries, some members stressed the value of the reciprocity of friendships: 'paying attention to needs of others was a healing experience' (Son et al. 2007: 96). Many older people are involved in volunteering for precisely this reason, because it is by its nature reciprocal. The Time Bank Scheme in the UK is an excellent example of how, through engaging in activities that involve supporting others as well as receiving support themselves, older people can increase their sense of self-worth, empowerment and self-confidence, as seen by this quote:

> I was very depressed and my GP encouraged me to join the Time Bank. I received time credits befriending an elderly lady who was blind, hosting barbecues and teaching English. When I was sick myself, I asked the time bank for help and they arranged meals and shopping for me. I also used my time credits to get my shed fixed. I've traveled to other time banks in London, to tell them my story.

(2005: 30)

---

**Box 6.2** Arts project combating social isolation

**Good times: art for older people at Dulwich Picture Gallery**

Dulwich Picture Gallery was awarded 'Highly Commended' in the Charity Awards 2006 for a project focused specifically on isolated older people.

The Gallery had spent several months researching isolation among older people. They found that: over a third of people over 65 live alone; seven in ten women over 85 live alone; over 25 per cent of people over 60 say they have no best friend, and 32 older people die alone and unnoticed every day.

As a result of this research, the Gallery devised a number of pilot schemes with local health services, social services and the voluntary sector to see what they could offer to isolated groups and individuals. The most common views on how isolation could be reduced involved activities, help with transport and outings.

The Education Department either brings people to the Gallery – or goes to them – and shows them round, talking to them about paintings. Most of the participants will never have been to an art gallery before. A most important part of the visit is tea followed by a practical art lesson.

(Adapted from: www.dulwichpicturegallery.org.uk/sackler/reaching_out/articles/25 7.aspx)

---

This case study illustrates an innovative way in which an arts project dealt with combating social isolation in a London community and indicates yet again the importance of friendships and access to activities for improving the well-being of vulnerable older people.

## Social and cognitive engagement

High levels of social engagement are a necessary part of successful ageing (Rowe and Khan 1997). Therefore, the need to support older people to explore satisfactory social activities remains an important part of promoting mental health and well-being (see Chapter 7). Engagement in social networks can sustain independence and choice for older people and provide a buffer against negative aspects of ageing and their impact on mental health and well-being (Bowling et al. 2002; Keller-Cohen et al. 2006; Clemence 2006; Son et al. 2007; Hutchison et al. 2008). The evidence, however, from a number of studies suggests it is the quality of the relationship as opposed to the quantity of relationships that is important (Wenger 1994; Moriarty and Butt 2004; Victor et al. 2005).

Some studies have found a relationship between social interactions and cognitive ability in later life. Less cognitive decline has been associated with more diverse social networks, greater engagement in community activities and greater emotional support (Bassuk et al. 1999; Seeman et al. 2001; Zenzunegui et al. 2003). Social engagement was found to be a protective element in preventing cognitive decline and retaining language skills (Keller-Cohen et al. 2006). Increased opportunities for older people to re-engage with society, and create and develop positive relationships, need to be a priority for policy-makers, health and social care staff as well as older people.

# Factors that impact on the formation of relationships

A number of environmental and social factors impact on an older person's ability to engage with and maintain a wide social network. These factors include demographic and social variables, gender, culture, disability and ageism.

## Demographic and social variables

Evidence indicates some class difference in what are seen as important relationships in older age. Research shows how demographic and economic status tends to determine network type, for example, middle-class older people who are more highly educated tend to establish relationships more quickly, and turn to friends for help rather than family. Working-class people, on the other hand, tend to have smaller kin-dominated networks in which the mother–daughter relationship is often especially strong (Wenger 1992). As we have seen earlier, different types of social networks offer varying support to older people. The relevance of these different networks to an older person's well-being allows health professionals to identify when an older person's social network provides a strong protective mechanism for supporting well-being and when it may not. It suggests that those with networks that are primarily focused on nearby kin with limited wider social networks may be particularly vulnerable.

   A lack of transport options may increase social isolation, restricting the ability to leave the house or for family and friends to visit easily. Equally, moving to a care home can present problems for friends and family, especially if they are reliant on public transport to visit (Cotteril and Taylor 2001). Furthermore, the forced reliance on public transport, for example, when an older person has to give up driving, may affect their sense of control over their life and thus diminish their self-esteem and sense of well-being. However, this may not necessarily be the case; Holland et al. (2005) reported that some people found travelling by public transport to be a positive experience providing them with an opportunity to meet and interact with others.

## Gender

The research on relationships in older people suggests that men's experience differs in some ways from women's. Men are less likely to have extensive networks in older age, and women more likely to maintain close relationships with same sex friends (Wenger 1992). For current generations of older people, men are likely to have more occupational attachments while women, who have typically had different patterns of employment and possibly less reliance on work-based friendships, may be better equipped to adjust to retirement or other major life events.

In a study by Davidson et al. (2005) the sample of men were more likely to have an extended network if they were married, although this was mainly as a result of the wife's network. The married men also reported helping widowed friends and neighbours, but again this was mainly at the instigation of the wife. If the wife died, men were less likely to maintain their wide social network, and became more focused on children and siblings for their emotional and instrumental support (Davidson et al. 2005). The experience of widowhood also differs for men and women with a greater per centage of men living with their partner until death (Higgs et al. 2004). One study found widowed men were three times more likely to commit or think about committing suicide than their married counterparts and that the first 12 months after being widowed presented the greatest risk (O'Connell et al. 2004). This suggests that marriage may offer some protection against suicide.

Older people who become isolated and lonely are at greater risk of suffering from depression and this in turn increases the risk of suicide (O'Connell et al. 2008). Gender differences feature strongly in relation to suicide among older people. In Western societies the incidence of completed suicides is three to four times more likely in men than women (Cattell 2000; O'Connell et al. 2004). However, in a study comparing Asian and English-speaking countries, while overall rates were similar, the incidence of suicide was greater in women in Asian societies (Pritchard and Baldwin 2002). This higher suicide rate among women was also found in Chinese rural areas and may in part be explained by changing socio-cultural pressures, which are tending to see less emphasis on the value and wisdom of older people. This may be experienced as a loss of status and give rise to feelings of hopelessness and uselessness often expressed by older people prior to suicide (Pritchard and Baldwin 2002). Another gender difference was found in older people with serious physical health problems, especially visual impairment, neurological disorders, and malignant disease, where older men were found to be more vulnerable to the risk of suicide than women (Waern et al. 2002; O'Connell et al. 2004).

## Culture

Culture, particularly religious tradition, exerts a strong influence on well-being among older people. A study exploring quality of life (Higgs et al. 2004) found that religion among older people from many ethnic minority communities was a strong provider of emotional support in times of stress. Religious belief helped the individual maintain a sense of self, identity and continuity, and thus reinforced positive well-being. Similarly, a study of African American elders (Jang et al. 2006) found the more traditional the group, the more positive the impact of religion on their mental well-being. Likewise, a study of 83 Latino elders (Beyenne et al. 2002) found that strong religious beliefs contributed to a sense of well-being.

Cultural expectations relating to one's family and community are also important markers in terms of mental health and well-being. The quality of social support and how well cultural expectations were met were important factors in the study of

Latino elders (Beyenne et al. 2002). In a survey on loneliness in an older population in China, living in a rural area and/or feeling that children were no longer showing filial piety were positive indicators of loneliness (Yang and Victor 2008). Because filial piety is so strongly embedded in Chinese culture the anxiety over family not fulfilling their obligations was increasingly linked not only with feelings of 'loss of face' but also anxiety they might be destitute and abandoned in old age. In the same study, females over the age of 85, especially those who were single or widowed, reported the highest levels of loneliness. This is not dissimilar to Western countries but, in addition, those Chinese living in rural areas reported significantly higher levels of loneliness compared to their urban counterparts (Yang and Victor 2008).

### Disability

Deteriorating health, loss of sight or hearing, increased fear and risk of falls, and reduced mobility can disrupt relationships, and are major contributors to loneliness and social isolation. Disability not only affects the older person's ability to engage in social interactions but also reduces the number of people with whom they might expect to come into contact. As one woman put it: 'As my hearing deteriorated I really missed having a conversation with people when I went shopping, or with neighbours. I began to feel really left out' (SEU 2005: 35).

Older people with sight and/or hearing loss are often unable to participate fully in their social environment. Embarrassment at not hearing or seeing well enough to engage with peers or social networks can leave the older person feeling isolated and withdrawn. If these impairments are not dealt with adequately the older person may become depressed (Cooke 2007).

### Ageism

Ageist attitudes persist in society and can profoundly affect relationships between older people and other generations. If the public generally tends towards a negative view of ageing, then individual interactions with older people are likely to be mediated by this view and this, in turn, can impact negatively on the older person's sense of well-being. As Edwards and Chapman suggest, 'ageist attitudes and assumptions permeate interpersonal interactions and communication in gerontology and by doing so ageism becomes a barrier to promoting mental wellness' (2004: 18).

## Types of relationships

### Family

Relationships with spouses and children are seen as highly advantageous to supporting older people's mental health and well-being. According to Bostock and Millar's (2003) survey, family and friends were felt to be an important contributor to a sense of self and well-being in later life. Respondents reported a sense of pride and achievement in seeing their children do well as adults, as if in some way their children's achievements were a reflection on 'their own life's purpose'. However, they also reported that relationships within families were not always positive, as families could be overprotective, geographically distant, have mental health or other problems that resulted in stress and worry for the older person. Family relationships are very complex, and while for many they contribute positively to well-being by enhancing a sense of value, continuity and self-worth, this is not always the case. Relationships with family can also be negative for older people, and in some extreme instances can lead to abuse of the vulnerable older person. The burden of care giving can also place enormous stress on a relationship leading to loneliness, depression and anxiety.

It could be argued that there is a greater sense of duty and responsibility, and a lack of emotional engagement in family relationships, as the focus is more on the provision of instrumental rather than emotional support. This is the 'doing' part of a relationship, rather than the 'being'. 'Family relationships may have a negative effect on well-being if they are absent, but when present their obligatory nature means they are less likely than friendships to make a positive contribution to well-being' (Keller-Cohen et al. 2006: 599). If the support the older person receives is based on a sense of duty, it is likely to lead to tension in the relationship and a greater risk of the older person experiencing a negative impact on their well-being (Jerrome and Wenger 1999; Hutchison et al. 2008; Son et al. 2007). This may go some way to explaining why many older people report the support of friends as providing a greater impact on their well-being than that of family.

Despite this, families continue to contribute to the positive well-being of many older people as they move through the transitions of later life. Jerrome and Wenger (1999) suggest that as people reach late old age and friendships begin to fade, through death or geographical relocation, the importance of children and siblings increases. Whereas, in early retirement, older people often rely on friends for their social support, as they age and become more dependent, they rely more on family and instrumental care.

*Cultural expectations*

A study in Buenos Aires looked at the life history of 22 men and women living in an area of high social deprivation, focusing on the impact of parent–child relationships on participants' well-being (Lloyd-Sherlock and Locke 2008). This study challenges some of the existing assumptions about the level of support older people receive from their family in developing countries. The authors argued that 'social change and economic instability have put families under growing strain, to the particular detriment of women's well-being' (Lloyd-Sherlock and Locke 2008: 783). Many older participants in the study felt resentful at the lack of support and help they received from their children or grandchildren, and this had a negative impact on their sense of self and well-being. Despite this many of the participants reframed their children's neglect in a more positive light with comments such as 'they have to look after their own family' or 'the neighbourhood is too dangerous for visiting'.

Although stereotypes of supportive extended families remain prevalent, the research literature increasingly highlights the shifting patterns of family support in developing countries. In a Chinese study (Yang and Victor 2008), socio-economic change affecting family structures led to some older people reporting concerns about children not fulfilling their duty. This caused them to experience a greater degree of depression and anxiety as they felt let down by their children.

## Friends

A number of studies have explored the meaning of friendships in the lives of older people and what it is about these friendships that is important to their mental health and well-being. The positive value of seeking social contact of a certain quality for successful ageing is highlighted in the two studies exploring the value of participation in an organization such as the Red Hat Society (see the case study in Box 6.3) (Son et al. 2007; Hutchison et al. 2008). Developing and maintaining friendships was found to support the development of self, self-confidence and self-esteem. Members of the Society reported a number of positive impacts on well-being, including opportunities for developing and strengthening friendships that provided the support necessary to deal with and manage a variety of stressors in their lives, including the loss of loved ones and the pressures of caring (Son et al. 2007; Hutchison et al. 2008). Membership also gave a shared sense of identity which is known to contribute to well-being. It has been suggested that the structure and purpose of the Red Hat Society with its emphasis on fun, playfulness and creativity may have specific benefits in improving older women's mental health and well-being, and that mainstream services such as day services, leisure clubs, etc., could learn from it. Although membership of the Red Hat Society was from a fairly homogenous group of white middle-class women and its claims have not been fully evaluated, nevertheless it underlines the value placed on friendships for support in coping with the many transitions of older age.

---

**Box 6.3** The Red Hat Society

The importance of fun and opportunities for developing supportive and reciprocal friendships is illustrated in the case of the Red Hat Society. It was started in America by Sue Ellen Cooper who was inspired by the poem *Warning* by Jenny Joseph – 'When I am old I will wear purple'. It offers women over 50 years of age in over 30 countries an opportunity to join a sisterhood of like-minded women motivated by the idea of having fun. There are now over 40,000 chapters of the Red Hat Society throughout the world. The first chapters were set up in the United Kingdom about seven years ago. Currently there are nearly 80 chapters across the UK, and everyone is welcome to join or to set up their own chapter.

A study by Son et al. (2007) of the Red Hat Society in America analysed 1693 responses from an online survey of members and found that older people reported their lives had been enriched, citing 'multiple psychosocial health benefits from their participation in the Red Hat Society ... creating happy moments, responding to transitions and negative events, and enhancing the self' (Son et al. 2007: 89).

Reflect on how this type of society might be helpful to the older women you know and would the same approach work for men?

A longitudinal study looking at friendships in people over 80 years of age found that even in late old age friendships were not static (Jerrome and Wenger 1999). The findings suggest that while some friendships fade, others are developed to take their place. This study highlights the importance of supporting older people to engage in opportunities for making new friendships as well as maintaining existing ones.

## Confiding relationships

Another dimension of social relationships relates to the presence of specific close relationships with people in whom one can confide. Such relationships are qualitatively different from other friendships and may perhaps be characterized as 'personal' rather than 'social'. Research indicates that older couples living together are more likely to view each other as confidants, whereas those living on their own often reported close friends as confidants rather than family members (Wenger 1994). A study in 1992 of older people in China found that 47.7 per cent identified their spouse as their confidant; 26.3 per cent identified a daughter; 19.6 per cent identified a son; and only 10.2 per cent identified friends and neighbours (Yang and Victor 2008). These results may relate to the expectations of the role of family in relation to the concepts of filial piety in this cohort of Chinese older people rather than a more general picture of older people.

While a confiding relationship may be with a spouse or other family member, frequently it will be with a close friend. Having friends, particularly a confidant, is important for self-image, well-being, mental health and the prevention of loneliness (Bowling et al. 2002). Wenger (1992) showed that the presence of a confidant within the network of relationships is linked with morale. Moriarty and Butt (2004) found that satisfaction with support levels was related to the quality of two or more confiding relationships rather than to the number of contacts with members of their family, friends or neighbours. These studies argue that having one or more confidant, either family or friends, has several positive outcomes including a sense of self, identity and self-worth, protection against loneliness and social isolation, opportunities for mutual support, shared experiences and having fun. These have been found to provide buffers to the negative effects of life events and associated stress on well-being (Bowling et al. 2002; Clemence 2006; Keller-Cohen et al. 2006; Son et al. 2007; Hutchison et al. 2008). They also point out the importance of same generation friends, which are more difficult to maintain as people grow older.

## Relationships with formal carers

With increasing age and frailty, many older people come to rely on carers to support them to continue living in the community or to care for them in a residential care setting. Older people frequently talk about the importance of developing a good relationship with those caring for them. The quality of the care environment and the way professional/paid care staff perceive their role, as well as the choices they afford older people, have a direct impact on the well-being and quality of life of older people.

Health and social care professionals are in an ideal position to promote mental well-being in their older clients. However, studies suggest that interactions are often focused on the physical and technical aspects of the task, with staff employing 'interpersonal control strategies' (Edwards and Chapman 2004: 17). This consists of giving directions and not enabling the older person to participate in decisions over their care, thus reinforcing a sense of dependency rather than promoting independence. For interactions to have a positive impact on an older person's mental health and well-being, the professional/care worker needs to demonstrate that they are listening and hearing what the person is saying. This requires all staff working with older people to challenge their own interpersonal skills, recognizing the inherent inequality in their encounters with vulnerable older people and ensuring the 'content of any conversation will not be directive, controlling or delivered in words more suitable for a young child rather than an older adult' (Edwards and Chapman 2004: 20). The use of life stories and narratives enable staff to learn to know and value the older person they are working with, which in turn helps the person to feel valued and listened to, and enhances the reciprocal nature of the interaction.

## Intimate relationships

Intimate relationships in later life provide the older person with a number of positive outcomes enhancing mental health and well-being. Intimacy and sexuality are often interlinked in the literature in relation to older people. Intimacy, however, is much more than just the sexual act of intercourse; it is about feelings of closeness, sharing of experiences, touch and recognition of mutual needs, affection and friendliness, companionship, physical nearness, a sense of belonging and self-identity (Garrett 1994). These are all elements which go into the experience of human intimacy and friendships and are essential for any age and any sexual orientation. As one author suggests, sexuality is about 'those ways of behaving which enrich the personality and enhance the relationships between people' (Grigg 1999: 12). Having an intimate relationship, whether it be with husband or wife, partners of differing sex or same sex, it is clear that individuals derive many benefits from the relationship.

Society often sees older people as asexual and unlikely to derive the same pleasure from a sexual experience as someone younger. This is especially true for gay, lesbian and bisexual older people who largely remain a hidden sub-group among older people (Harris and Weir 1998; Ward et al. 2005). Evidence challenges this stereotypical view of ageing and suggests that older people are as likely as younger people to experience the positive benefits of sexuality and to remain sexually active. A Swedish study of people aged over 70 (Persson 1980) found that those who were sexually active reported a number of positive outcomes to health and well-being: men were found to sleep better, be more mentally active and have a more positive attitude to sexuality in old age; women retained their former levels of emotional stability, had lower levels of anxiety and reported feeling physically and mentally healthier.

While sexuality may have a positive impact on mental health and well-being, the loss of an intimate partner, whether heterosexual or homosexual, is likely to have a negative impact on mental health and well-being, often leading to depression or in some cases suicide. The importance of sustaining the intimate relationships of all older people and providing support mechanisms when someone loses a partner through death, separation or divorce needs to be recognized.

*Same sex relationships*

Gott (2005) suggests that there is a tendency to regard older people as heterosexual despite the fact that about 10 per cent of the population is not heterosexual and that older people are, clearly, represented in that group. The result is that 'the lived experience of gay, lesbian and bisexual older people is missing from research policy and practice' (Gott 2005: 124). Consequently relatively little is known about the nature of dating and intimacy as it evolves over time in the relationships of older homosexual men and women. Although older homosexual men and women experience the same bodily changes with ageing and the same emotions as older heterosexual people, they may also face unique challenges, such as the loss of a partner through HIV infection, a higher risk of social isolation and, if the older person experiences ill health, they and their partners may be subject to negative attitudes by health professionals. Equally, a number of gay, lesbian and bisexual older people may have difficulty disclosing their sexuality to health care providers for fear of stigma and prejudice. Several organizations now support the older homosexual community. Those older people living in gay and lesbian communities are more likely to have a wide network of support relationships, whereas those living in the wider community may be more isolated with a smaller and less diverse network of support (Ward 2000; Ward et al. 2005). Strategies need to be developed to support gay, lesbian and bisexual older people to express their sexuality and to receive the support they need from health and social services.

## Intergenerational relationships: grandparenting

Chapter 7 deals with broad intergenerational activities in the context of social activities to promote mental health and well-being. Here we will focus specifically on the intergenerational relationship of grandparenting, recognizing that much of the research applies equally to other important relationships that older people have with younger people, for example, with god-children, the children of friends or siblings, etc. Estimates by Age Concern suggest 29 per cent of the adult population in the UK experience grandparenthood with three-quarters of those being over 65 years of age. The numbers in the USA are similar, suggesting that the grandparent/grandchild relationship may have an important role in promoting mental health and well-being in around one-third of older people (Harper 2005).

Over the last decade there has been increased interest from policy-makers, campaigners and researchers on the role of grandparenting and the relationship between grandparents and grandchildren (Bullock 2001; Clarke and Roberts 2004; Clarke et al. 2005; Broad 2007). Although there is greater recognition of the importance of grandparents and their role supporting families to remain together, or remain economically viable by caring for grandchildren while the parents work, governments still fail to provide adequate resources for grandparents to take on this supporting role. Safeguarding the interests of grandparents and ensuring access in the event of marital breakdown are also priorities.

### Meaning of grandparenthood

The grandparent/grandchild role not only has emotional ties but is also seen as symbolic in promoting continuity of the older person's gene pool: 'I feel as if compared to work I've achieved something ... I've used my time usefully and they are kind of like the end product' (Clarke and Roberts 2004: 201). This sense of continuity and pride in grandchildren is also highlighted in the sense of well-being expressed by participants in a study from minority ethnic groups, who saw grandchildren and their behaviour as a reflection on themselves within their community (Nazroo et al. 2004).

In an in-depth study of 45 older grandparents Clarke and Roberts (2003) identified three types of support grandparents provided: practical, financial and emotional. However, the degree of each type of support varied depending on the grandparent/grandchild relationship. The global nature of family life may mean the older person has little contact with grandchildren. Nonetheless, this study found that three in five grandparents saw at least one grandchild on a weekly basis and that 64 per cent lived in close proximity to their grandchild. They also reported other contact via email and phone calls, and the majority of grandparents in the study reported receiving high levels of satisfaction and enjoyment from these interactions. Geographical proximity to grandchildren clearly played a large part in determining frequency of contact. There was also some variation in levels of contact between paternal or maternal grandparents; grandparents were less likely to see grandchildren if they were paternal grandparents and their son had separated (Clarke and Roberts 2004).

### Grandparenting roles

In many studies older people report that being a grandparent enables reciprocity and provides a fulfilling role. Some older men report that they enjoy looking after their grandchildren as it gives them the opportunities they may not have had when their own children were growing up. Others talked about the role keeping them 'young at heart' and up to date. For some it provided a reason for getting up in the morning, a sense of fulfilment and of being a valued member of society as well as helping family (Clarke and Roberts 2004: Nazroo et al. 2004; Clarke et al. 2005; Broad 2007).

A study by Nazroo et al. (2004) looking at the role older people played as grandparents in four different ethnic groups (Jamaican Caribbean, Gujarati Indian

Hindu, Punjabi Pakistani and White English) found some variation by gender and ethnicity in the way these roles were experienced. For older people living in multigenerational families, many take on the role of carer for the grandchildren while the parents go out to work. This is particularly true for older women who continue to provide the nurturing role they provided for their own children. Older Gujarati and Punjabi Pakistani elders, especially men, saw their role with their grandchildren as a way of retaining and passing on the culture and religion of their forefathers.

The arrival of grandchildren is universally celebrated, but the experience of grandparenting differs according to individual circumstances, culture and socio-economic factors. Its potential to impact positively and negatively on mental health will vary as the following case studies illustrate.

---

**Box 6.4** Case studies: mental health and grandparenting

### Case study A

Jane, a widow, retired five years ago hoping to develop new interests, visit friends and maybe find a new partner. Her daughter, who has three children, divorced two years ago and works full-time. Jane looks after the children, two not yet in school. She loves them greatly but finds the caring and level of responsibility very tiring. She would like to spend more time with other people in the day, but doesn't feel very welcome at parent and toddler groups and her friends don't want small children around for long. She knows others are in a similar situation to her and thinks she ought to start up some support activities. She feels increasingly isolated and often unhappy.

### Case study B

Kate and Steve are in their late 60s and have four grandchildren. None live nearby so visits are anticipated with great pleasure. Seeing the children grow and develop is a highlight of their lives. Both feel good when their skills in planning fun activities are received with such pleasure. The earlier experience of bringing up their own children has made them relaxed about the different ways that the grandchildren develop and confident in making them feel secure. Occasionally they look after the children for weekends which is enjoyable but tiring. They sometimes feel anxious about the nature of childhood in the twenty-first century and worry about some of the challenges the children will face.

*Pressures of grandparenting*

As the case studies above demonstrate, grandparents are increasingly being recognized as a group able to take on the care of grandchildren when there are pressures on families or a breakdown of family networks. In especially vulnerable families grandparents may also be well placed to protect their grandchildren from abuse. While for some being a very active grandparent can have a positive impact on well-being, for others it can be negative, placing a far greater burden of responsibility on the older person than they would wish. One older man suggested that while he valued the relationship with his granddaughter sufficiently to take over her care, he felt it was 'like, putting your life on hold, you know, for what is going to be ten, fifteen years, I don't know' (Clarke et al. 2005: 68).

In the same study other grandparents reported a negative impact, having children and grandchildren return home after a marriage failure or some other major crisis. While the impact was not immediate, over time it could affect their well-being. The degree of worry they felt and the restrictions this change had on their own activities could lead to feelings of negative well-being and in some cases depression (Clarke et al. 2005). In cases where the older person had been forced to take on a more involved role such as adopting or caring for grandchildren, this could have a negative impact on well-being both emotionally and financially.

*Grandparents as surrogate parents*

In many African and Asian communities the AIDS pandemic means that many older people, especially women, find themselves not only caring for their children as they die, but also caring for their orphaned grandchildren. In 2006, HelpAge International estimated that between 40 and 60 per cent of orphans in a number of Sub-Saharan countries were living in grandmother-headed households (www.helpage.org). Many older people were already caring for their grandchildren within a reciprocal relationship where older adults were working in the cities and providing financial support to the grandmothers and children. What has changed with AIDS is that the reciprocal relationship has broken down and grandmothers, as well as caring for their orphaned grandchildren have also become the main breadwinner, being forced to work in order to feed themselves and their family (Chazan 2008). Many older people in these countries now experience a decline in status, financial and emotional hardship, loss of respect and untreated chronic illness, leading to an increased sense of vulnerability and the lack of well-being (see the case study in Box 6.5) (Knodel and VanLandingham 2002; Oppong 2006; Knodel 2005; Chazan 2008).

**Box 6.5** Surrogate parenthood: a case study

**What needs to be done to support Miriam?**

Miriam's income comes from selling produce from her smallholding. Two of her children and their partners have died from HIV AIDS and she is bringing up their five children. To lose her own children was a great shock and sadness but she had little time to grieve. Fulfilling her responsibilities for her grandchildren has placed strains on her. She is less strong than she was, her income has dropped and she worries about keeping the grandchildren in school. What would happen to them if she died is her biggest anxiety. Many of her friends are in a similar situation and they give each other support but are usually too exhausted in the evenings to do anything but sleep. She misses their singing and storytelling and often feels sad and rather lonely.

Question: What needs to be done to support Miriam?

The evidence presented here illustrates the complexity of the grandparent/ grandchild relationship and the role it plays in promoting positive well-being in older people. It highlights the need for governments nationally and internationally to look more carefully at policies and services, as well as making the role more visible to the policy and research communities in order to support older people in fulfilling their role with grandchildren (Broad 2007).

## Strategies for promoting mental health and well-being

The promotion of mental health and well-being has been discussed throughout the chapter and a number of themes have emerged which may be helpful for older people and those working with them to provide services and care to enhance positive well-being.

### Policy and practice

The problem of loneliness and social isolation and its negative impact on well-being is recognized in a number of policy initiatives (DH 1999 and 2001; WHO 2002; SEU 2005). However, there has been little evidence of the effectiveness of such initiatives to date. In 2005 a systematic review was undertaken to evaluate the 'effectiveness of health promotion interventions that target loneliness and social isolation in older people' (Cattan et al. 2005: 41). The review explored a number of group and one-to-one interventions and found that educational and social activity in groups demonstrated some effectiveness in preventing loneliness and social isolation, whereas the evidence for strategies aimed at one-to-one activities, such as befriending, was less conclusive (Cattan et al. 2005). This systematic review begins to untangle some of the indicators for promoting mental health and well-being, but further research needs to be undertaken especially with one-to-one interventions, to see how services can be developed to provide effective mental health promotion.

In the section on grandparenting above, the evidence suggests there is still a need to address policies and resources to support older people in the crucial roles they play in their relationships with grandchildren. Structures are needed for those grandparents who have, as a result of family dysfunction or breakdown, become the primary or sole carer.

## Increasing community access and reducing social isolation

The following strategies are important in supporting older people to maintain positive social networks:

1   To improve access to social networks *better systems of public transport* are needed. A recent study (Marsden et al. 2007) looked at the importance of transport to older people and involved them in identifying solutions to the problems they experience. Key recommendations from this study include the need for better information about public transport, better access to mainstream transport and more segregated, high quality pedestrian areas. The researchers suggest 'there is an urgent need for major change in the planning and delivery of transport infrastructure and services so that older people's views are heard and their needs taken into account' (Marsden et al. 2007: 55).

2   Older people with *hearing and visual problems* are at risk of social isolation and poor mental health including loneliness and depression as they withdraw from relationships and activities in which they can no longer engage. Improved systems for assessment and provision of hearing aids and glasses, better environmental adaptations for older people with hearing and vision impairment, a greater public awareness of the importance of communicating, and working with those older people who have become excluded because of hearing and vision problems will go some way to overcoming these barriers.

3   Strategies to increase *the use of the Internet* for older people include the work being done by Age Concern's Silver Surfer networks. According to current statistics, only about 15 per cent of older people use the Internet (Age Concern England 2008). This number needs to be increased significantly so that older people can benefit from the positive impact it can bring to their mental health, especially older people who are socially isolated and housebound. It has the potential for older people to remain in contact with friends and family, develop new interests and hobbies, belong to online groups and chat rooms which provide opportunities for developing new relationships, and engaging in community action campaigns by having their say on issues which are important to them. The Silver Surfer project aims to increase access for older people to use the web but more focus needs to be on those who are confined to their home, for whatever reason, and who are unable to access the training provided by Age Concern Centres.

## Supporting social networks

To promote mental health and well-being individuals need to feel empowered and have a sense of self-efficacy. Relationships play a crucial role in this by supporting these attributes. Ability in later life is said to be enhanced by continued social interaction and perceived social support (Edwards and Chapman 2004). Interventions that are aimed at preventing isolation and loneliness as well as increasing self-worth and integration back into the community will also help alleviate depression and prevent suicide. Granted the fact that older people continue to replace lost friendships (Jerome and Wenger 1999), there is much that health and social care professionals working with older people can do to encourage and facilitate the development and maintenance of relationships. Here we have cited some examples of these such as the Time Bank Scheme and the Red Hat Society, and there are many more. Further research will be valuable to tease out the attributes inherent in these social groups that have such a positive impact on participants' well-being. Schemes which promote the skills and independence of older people are important for increasing well-being and social relationships.

A lot of the evidence from older people highlights the value they place on good interpersonal skills in supporting and developing positive interactions within their social care networks. Emphasis needs to be placed on the interactions of formal carers with older people, promoting good communication and underlining the need for a reciprocal relationship to be developed. This will enable the older person to feel confident and competent in their interactions with health and social care professionals.

Other interventions include better identification of severe depressive illness and greater support to people in the first 12 months following bereavement. A study of a sample of African Americans also found 'religiosity and life satisfaction' were independent protective factors against suicide and thoughts of suicide, and a further study of people with terminal illness found that 'higher spiritual well-being and life satisfaction also predicted lower suicidal feelings' (O'Connell et al. 2004: 898). Together with interventions to enhance psychological well-being, we need to increase interventions at population level that improve social contact, support and increase social capital in all older people.

## Recognizing the value of older people and challenging ageism

The need to challenge ageist stereotypes remains a pressing challenge as these can directly or inadvertently influence public service planning and delivery, and impact negatively on individuals' mental health and well-being. Activities and interventions that promote the value of older people are part of this challenge and are crucial to supporting a sense of self and empowerment on the part of older people themselves.

# Conclusion

The promotion of mental health in later life presents important challenges to society in general, and to health and social care professionals who work with older people in particular. Thus the focus of this chapter has been on one of the crucial components of good mental health and well-being – the ability to make and sustain relationships. Relationships that are both rich and stable provide a buffer against the feelings of anxiety, loneliness, depression and unhappiness, which are inclined to come with the lifestyle changes inherent in the ageing process.

However, the maintenance of established relationships and the creation of new ones become more difficult as people age. This is due in large part to their reducing ability to access social networks, deteriorating health and increasing disability, commitments to housebound partners, and ageist and cultural attitudes. This chapter has identified some of the policies and practices that encourage and enable older people to maintain and re-engage in activities which sustain and extend their social networks. Health and social professionals have an important role to play to ensure that these issues are addressed.

Certain attributes in an older person's relationships are particularly important to the maintenance of a positive sense of self and self-identity. Relationships which support and encourage positive attitudes enable older people to adapt to the transitions and changes in their lives. Relationships which allow the older person to give as well as receive help prevent the negative feelings which can arise from their increasing dependence on others. When an older person feels valued as an equal partner in the relationship, then their sense of dignity and self-worth is not diminished by the acceptance of care. Finally, relationships which have a high level of social interaction are associated with the maintenance of cognitive acuity and language skills, thus enabling the older person to remain in control of their lives.

Throughout our lives, we form many different types of relationships and the ones that are considered particularly important to older people have been discussed in this chapter. Family and friends rate very highly, however, there are some relationships unique to the older person, such as those with grandchildren and carers that also need to be recognized and supported. Older people need confidants with whom they can share their cares and concerns, but they frequently face the loss of these close relationships. Intimate relationships are important for older people but are often overlooked. Thus this chapter looked at sexual relationships as often being important components in the maintenance of a positive sense of self and self-identity.

Promoting mental health in later life provides an important challenge for society and one which needs to be taken seriously. To promote mental health and well-being it is essential that both policy and practice focus on enabling the voice of older people to influence future developments. As Jerrome and Wenger's (1999) study demonstrated, social networks of older people are not static, and continue to change depending on circumstances even into late old age. Health and social care professionals can encourage and support people to participate in activities that create opportunities for increasing social networks and making new friends. They can challenge ageist attitudes and work to support older people to become active participants in their communities, and empower them to have an effective role within family and community networks.

# Reflective questions

1 How can we challenge ageism and ensure that older people are able to maintain and develop intimate relationships regardless of sexual orientation?
2 What support mechanisms should we put in place to support grandparents when they need to take on the role of caring for grandchildren?
3 Think about who you would turn to for emotional support and why. Then ask some older people you know or work with the same question and compare answers.
4 Reflect on why it is that in Asian societies older women are more likely to commit suicide than men.
5 How can you support the relationships of the older people you know or work with?

# References

AC (Audit Commission) (2008) *Don't Stop Me Now*. London: Audit Commission.

Age Concern England (2008) Age Concern project aims put Silver Surfers online. Available at: www.brandrepublic.com/news/179797/ (accessed 8 Oct. 2008).

Bassuk, S., Glass, T. and Berkman, L. (1999) Social disengagement and incident cognitive decline in community-dwelling elderly persons, *Annals of Internal Medicine*, 131: 165–73.

Beyenne, Y., Becker, G. and Mayer, N. (2002) Perceptions of ageing and a sense of well-being among Latino elderly, *Journal of Cross-Cultural Gerontology*, 17(2): 155–72.

Bostock, Y. and Millar, C. (2003) *Older People's Perception of the Factors that Affect Mental Well-Being in Later Life*. Edinburgh: NHS Scotland.

Bowlby, J. (1988) *A Secure Base: Parent-Child Attachment and Healthy Human Development*. London: Routledge.

Bowling, A. (1995) 'What things are important in people's lives? A survey of the public's judgements to inform scales of health related quality of life', *Social Science and Medicine*, 41(10): 1447–62.

Bowling, A. (2005) *Ageing Well: Quality of Life in Old Age*. Maidenhead: Open University Press/McGraw-Hill.

Bowling, A., Banister, D. and Sutton, S. (2002) A multidimensional model of quality of life in older age, *Ageing and Mental Health*, 6: 355–71.

Broad, B. (2007) *Being a Grandparent: Research Evidence, Key Themes and Policy Recommendations*. Harlow: The Grandparents Association.

Bullock, K. (2001) The changing role of grandparents in rural America, *Education and Ageing*, 16(2): 163–78.

Cattan, M., Newell, C., Bond, J. and White, M. (2003) Alleviating social isolation and loneliness among older people, *International Journal of Mental Health Promotion*, 5(3): 20–30.

Cattan, M., White, M., Bond, J. and Learmouth, A. (2005) Preventing social isolation and loneliness among older people: a systematic review of health promotion interventions, *Ageing and Society*, 25(1): 41–67.

Cattell, H. (2000) Suicide in the elderly, *Advanced Psychiatric Treatment*, 6: 102–8.

Chazan, M. (2008) Seven 'deadly' assumptions: unravelling the implications of HIV/AIDS among grandmothers in South Africa and beyond, *Ageing & Society*, 28(7): 935–58.

Clarke, L., Evandrou, M. and Warr, P. (2005) Family and economic roles, in A. Walker (ed.) *Understanding Quality of Life in Old Age*. Maidenhead: Open University Press/McGraw-Hill.

Clarke, L. and Roberts, C. (2004) The meaning of grandparenthood and its contribution to the quality of life of older people, in A. Walker and C. Hennessey (eds) *Growing Older: Quality of Life in Old Age*. Maidenhead: Open University Press/McGraw-Hill.

Clemence, A., Karmaniola, A., Green, E. and Spini, D. (2007) Disturbing life events and well-being after 80 years of age: a longitudinal comparison of survivors and the deceased over five years, *Ageing and Society*, 27(2): 195–213.

Cotteril, L. and Taylor, D. (2001) Promoting mental health and well-being among housebound older people, *Quality in Ageing: Policy, Practice and Research*, 2(3): 29–43.

DH (Department of Health) (1999) *Saving Lives: Our Healthier Nation*. London: The Stationery Office.

DH (Department of Health) (2001) *National Service Framework for Older People*. London: The Stationery Office.

Edwards, H. and Chapman, H. (2004) Contemplating, caring, coping, conversing: a model for promoting wellness in later life, *Journal of Gerontological Nursing*, 30(5): 16–21.

Farquar, M. (1995) Elderly people's definition of quality of life, *Social Science and Medicine*, 41: 1439–46.

Fiori, K., Antonucci, A. and Akiyama, H. (2008) Profiles of social relations among older adults: a cross-cultural approach, *Ageing and Society*, 28(2): 203–31.

Garrett, G. (1994) Sexuality in later life, *Elderly Care*, 6(4): 23–8.

Gibson, H. (2001) Loneliness in later life, in A. Walker and C. Hennessy (eds) (2004) *Growing Older: Quality of Life in Old Age*. Maidenhead: Open University Press/McGraw-Hill.

Gott, M. (2005) *Sexuality, Sexual Health and Ageing*. Milton Keynes: Open University Press.

Grigg, E. (1999) Sexuality in older people, *Elderly Care*, 11(7): 12–15.

Harper, S. (2005) Grandparenthood, in M. Johnson in conjunction with V. Bengtson, P. Coleman and T. Kirkwood (eds) *The Cambridge Handbook of Age and Ageing*. Cambridge: Cambridge University Press.

Harris, L. and Weir, M. (1998) Inappropriate sexual behaviour in dementia: a review of the treatment literature, *Sexuality and Disability*, 16(3): 205–17.

Higgs, P., Hyde, M., Arber, S. et al. (2004) Dimensions of the inequalities in quality of life in older age, in A. Walker and C. Hennessy (eds) (2004) *Growing Older: Quality of Life in Old Age*. Maidenhead: Open University Press.

Holmen, K. and Fukurama, H. (2002) Loneliness, health and social network among elderly people: a follow-up study, *Archives of Gerontology and Geriatrics*, 53(3): 261–71.

Hutchison, S., Yarnal, C., Staffordson, J., and Kerstetter, D. (2008) Beyond fun and friendship: Red Hat Society as a coping resource for older women, *Ageing and Society*, 28(7): 979–99.

Jang, Y., Borenstein, A., Chirboga, D., Phillips, K. and Mortimer, J. (2006) Religiosity, adherence to tradition, culture, and psychological well-being among African American elders, *Journal of Applied Gerontology*, 25(5): 343–55.

Jerrome, D. and Wenger, C. (1999) Stability and change in later-life friendships, *Ageing and Society*, 19(6): 661–76.

Keller-Cohen, D., Fiori, K., Toler, A. and Bybee, D. (2006) Social relations, language and cognition in the 'oldest old', *Ageing and Society*, 26(4): 585–606.

Knodel, J. (2005) Researching the impact of the AIDS epidemic on older-age parents in Africa: lessons from studies in Thailand, *Generations Review*, 15(2): 16–22.

Knodel, J. and VanLandingham, M. (2002) The impact of the AIDS epidemic on older persons, *AIDS*, 16(Suppl. 3): S77–S83.

Litwin, H. (2001) Social network type and morale in old age, *Gerontologist*, 41(4): 516–24.

Lloyd-Sherlock, P. and Locke, C. (2008) Vulnerable relations: lifecourse, well-being and social exclusion in Buenos Aires, Argentina, *Ageing and Society*, 28(6): 779–803.

Marsden, G., Jopson, A., Cattan, M. and Woodward, J. (2007) *Transport and Older People: Integrating Transport Planning Tools with User Needs*. Leeds: University of Leeds / Leeds Metropolitan University. Available at: http://www.leedsmet.ac.uk/health/healthpromotion/chpr/projects/roadusers07.htm (accessed 18 Sept. 2008).

Moriarty, J. and Butt, J. (2004) Social support and ethnicity in old age, in A. Walker and C. Hennessey (eds) *Growing Older: Quality of Life in Old Age*. Maidenhead: Open University Press/McGraw-Hill.

Nazroo, J., Bajekal, M., Blane, D. and Grewal, I. (2004) Ethnic inequalities, in A. Walker and C. Hennessey (eds) *Growing Older: Quality of Life in Old Age*. Maidenhead: Open University Press/McGraw-Hill.

O'Connell, H., Chin, A., Cunningham, C. and Lawlor, B. (2004) Recent developments: suicide in older people, *British Medical Journal*, 329: 895–9.

Oppong, C. (2006) Familial roles and social transformations: older men and women in Sub-Saharan Africa, *Research on Ageing*, 28(6): 654–68.

Persson, G. (1980) Sexuality in a 70 year old urban population, *Journal of Psychosomatic Research*, 24: 335–42.

Pritchard, C. and Baldwin, D. (2002) Elderly suicide rates in Asian and English-speaking countries, *Acta Psychiatrica Scandinavia*, 105: 271–5.

Rowe, J. and Khan, R. (1997) Successful ageing, *Gerontologist*, 37(4): 433–40.

Seeman, T., Lusignolo, T., Albert, M. and Berkman, L. (2001) Social relationships, social support, and patterns of cognitive ageing in healthy, high functioning older adults: MacArthur studies of successful ageing, *Health Psychology*, 20(4): 243–55.

SEU (Social Exclusion Unit) (2005) *Excluded Older People*. London: Office of the Deputy Prime Minister.

Sheldon, J. (1948) The social medicine of old age, in A. Walker and C. Hennessy (eds) (2004) *Growing Older: Quality of Life in Old Age*. Maidenhead: Open University Press/McGraw-Hill.

Smith, A. (2000) *Researching Quality of Life of Older People: Concepts, Measures and Findings*. Working Paper No. 7. Keele: Centre for Social Gerontology Keele University.

Son, J., Kerstetter, D., Yarnal, C. and Baker, B. (2007) Promoting older people's health and well-being through social leisure environments: what we have learned from The Red Hat Society, *Journal of Women & Ageing*, 19: 89–104.

Townsend, P. (1968) Isolation and loneliness, in A. Walker and C. Hennessy (eds) (2004) *Growing Older: Quality of Life in Old Age*. Maidenhead: Open University Press/McGraw-Hill.

Victor, C. and Scharf, T. (2005) Social isolation and loneliness, in A. Walker (ed.), *Understanding Quality of Life in Old Age*. Maidenhead: Open University Press/McGraw-Hill.

Victor, C., Scrambler, S., Bond, J. and Bowling, A. (2004) Loneliness in later life, in A. Walker and C. Hennessy (eds) *Growing Older: Quality of Life in Old Age*. Maidenhead: Open University Press/McGraw-Hill.

Victor, C., Scrambler, S., Bowling, A. and Bond, J. (2005) The prevalence of and risk factors for loneliness in later life: a survey of older people in Great Britain, *Ageing and Society*, 25(3): 357–75.

Victor, C., Scrambler, S., Shah, S. et al. (2002) Has loneliness among older people increased? An investigation into variations between cohorts, *Ageing and Society*, 22(1): 1–13.

Waern, M., Rubenowitz, E., Runeson, B. et al. (2002) Burden of illness and suicide in elderly people: case-control study, *British Medical Journal*, 324: 1355–8.

Walker, A. (ed.) (2005) *Understanding Quality of Life in Old Age*. Maidenhead: Open University Press/McGraw-Hill.

Walker, A. and Hennessy, C. (eds) (2004) *Growing Older: Quality of Life in Old Age*. Maidenhead: Open University Press/McGraw-Hill.

Ward, R. (2000) Waiting to be heard: dementia and the gay community, *Journal of Dementia Care*, 8(3): 24–5.

Ward, R., Vass, A., Aggarwal, N., Garfield, C. and Cybyk, B. (2005) A kiss is still a kiss? The construction of sexuality in dementia care, *DEMENTIA*, 4(1): 49–72.

Wenger, C. (1992) *Help in Old Age*, Institute of Human Ageing Occasional Papers No 5. Liverpool: Liverpool University Press.

Wenger, C. (1994) *Understanding Support Networks and Community Care*. Avebury: Aldershot.

Wenger, C. (1996) Social networks and gerontology, *Reviews in Clinical Gerontology*, 6: 285–93.

Wenger, C. (2000) How important is parenthood? Childlessness and support in old age, *Ageing and Society*, 20: 161–82.

WHO (World Health Organization) (2002) *Active Ageing: A Policy Framework*. Geneva: WHO.

Wilhelmson, K., Andersson, C., Waern, M. and Allebeck, P. (2005) Elderly people's perspectives on quality of life, *Ageing and Society*, 25(4): 585–600.

Wilson, G. (1994) Co-production and self-care: new approaches to managing community care services for older people, *Social Policy and Administration*, 28(3): 236–50.

Witzelben, H. (1968) On loneliness, *Psychiatry*, 21: 31–43.

Yang, K. and Victor, C. (2008) The prevalence of and risk factors for loneliness among older people in China, *Ageing and Society*, 28(3): 305–27.

Zenzunegui, M., Alvarado, B., Del Ser, T. and Otero, A. (2003) Social networks, social integration, and social engagement determine cognitive decline in community-dwelling Spanish older adults, *Journal of Gerontology: Social Sciences*, 58B(2): Z93–100.

# 7    Keeping active
## Angela Clow and Liz Aitchison

## Editor's foreword

This chapter considers the third theme identified by older people as important for their mental health, namely physical and mental activity. It starts by considering the theoretical framework for keeping active and reviewing recent policies that have promoted activity as a way of maintaining mental well-being in later life. The chapter is then divided into three clear sections: factors associated with physical activity and mental health, factors associated with mental activity and mental well-being, and, finally, a substantial section on evidence and theoretically based practice in these two areas. Importantly, this section demonstrates the wide range of areas where mental health promotion can have an impact on older people's health.

## Introduction

This chapter aims to explore the link between 'activity' and mental health and well-being in older people. Successful ageing has been described as multidimensional, involving the maintenance of high physical and cognitive function as well as sustained engagement in social and productive activities (Rowe and Kahn 2000). Accordingly we will explore three broad and interrelated themes. The first is the role of physical activity in promoting successful ageing. There is compelling evidence that regular physical activity by older people not only maintains strength and agility and decreases risk of physical illness (such as heart disease, diabetes and some cancers) but also has positive impacts on cognitive ability, mood and general well-being. So keeping physically active has replaced old notions that retirement is the time to 'put your feet up'. Second, we explore the evidence that mental or intellectual activity promotes well-being, improves quality of life and helps protect from cognitive decline. Third, we consider aspects of social activity – specifically activities that can broadly be seen as participation in society and between the generations. The World Health Organization (WHO 2002) has defined active ageing as having not only physical and psychological dimensions but also as the capacity to participate in society. Social and cultural activities have been shown to be beneficial in terms of well-being, functioning and survival (Glass et al. 1999). What is clear is that successful ageing involves a complex interplay between personal and social factors – however, a common feature is 'activity', be that physical, cognitive or social.

# Theoretical framework

Chapter 3 presents a full discussion of theoretical perspectives on ageing and health promotion, and several theories are relevant here, for example, continuity theory, social interactionist theory and activity theory. Equally, concepts such as empowerment, self-efficacy, resilience and environmental mastery have been shown to fundamentally influence mental health and well-being (see Chapters 2 and 3). Keeping physically and mentally active and continuing to participate in society can help to promote and sustain the sense of being in control of one's life.

The dramatic increase in life expectancy for people in developed countries has produced a substantial literature on the use of 'leisure' time in older age. Various theories about the leisure styles of retired people have developed, with research tending to focus on the relationship between certain activities and the demographic profile of older people taking part in them, and the psycho-social outcomes that result. Activity theory (Havighurst 1963) argues that in order to preserve mental well-being in old age it is important to keep involved in activities, maintaining the activities of middle age or finding substitutes. This replaced earlier theories of older age as a time of 'disengagement' or gradual withdrawal from society. Many studies have supported the contribution that high levels of involvement in activity make to mental and psychological well-being.

Baltes and Baltes (1990) asserted that it is healthy to adapt to the biological, mental and social changes that take place as one ages, and that this can be done by being selective about one's activities, dropping those that are less meaningful, or perhaps less manageable, and optimizing the rest. This was called 'selective optimization with compensation' (see Chapter 2) and, in further research using this approach (Janke and Davey 2004, in Nimrod and Adoni 2006), a decrease in depressive symptoms was shown.

However, investigation into the relationship between types of activity, mental health and well-being has been complicated by the problem of direction of causality – in other words, do happier, healthier people tend to participate in more activity or does the activity make people happier and healthier? This type of research is also complicated by the existence of associated lifestyle factors. For example, people who choose to exercise regularly may also eat a healthier diet and be more sociable than those who do not. These interrelationships often make it difficult to tease out the *'active ingredient'* in the promotion of successful ageing. More recently these problems have been addressed by powerful prospective studies which examine the impact of specific interventions (such as an exercise programme). In these types of studies it is possible to examine response in the variables of interest (e.g., mental health and well-being) over a period of time relative to an initial starting point and compared to groups of similar people not exposed to the intervention. Where possible we will review cross-sectional (where causality cannot be inferred) and prospective studies to provide evidence for the role of participation in activity in promoting well-being.

## Policy framework

The growing focus on remaining active has meant a shift away from the view that retirement is a time to sit back and take it easy. A new set of socio-cultural expectations about older age are influencing public policy. The implications of an ageing population and the associated costs of pensions and care are a major concern to policy-makers (see Chapters 2 and 4). Addressing the underlying determinants of health and well-being in older age is a priority and one would expect to see policy initiatives promoting physical activity. In the UK, policy in relation to older people and mental health and well-being is set out in two National Service Frameworks (NSF), the *National Service Framework for Older People* (DH 2001) and the *National Service Framework for Mental Health* (DH 1999). The former is predominantly focused on the treatment and management of the common diseases of older age (such as stroke), on prevention (such as falls) and on the mechanisms within the health care system (such as intermediate care) to support older people at risk of hospitalization. However, it does contain a chapter on the promotion of health and active life in older age, and urges health and local government bodies to work together to increase physical activity. While the overall aim is to delay frailty and disability, and to promote quality of life, no explicit focus on improving mental well-being is evident. Where this is mentioned, it is in the context of the management and treatment of mental illness such as depression and issues around the care of people with dementia. The advent of the NSF and of closer working between health and social care agencies and the voluntary sector has undoubtedly had a positive impact on the keeping active agenda, with a greater emphasis being given at a local level to initiatives that aim to engage older people in healthy activities, as evidenced by the wider range of activities available to older people in certain settings (see Table 7.1). The *National Service Framework for Mental Health* does not address older people specifically and the kinds of mental health promotion strategies that have flowed from this NSF have not tended to focus on older people as a target group. In contrast, older people are a priority in the Scottish programme *Improving Mental Health and Well-Being* (Scottish Executive 2003).

Policy relating to age and keeping active tends to be defined from the perspective of younger people, has a focus on physical health and disease prevention, and is articulated within a material framework evidenced by the language of productivity, income and public expenditure. From the perspective of older people themselves, an active life does not necessarily mean 'participating in the activity-driven goals of younger people, but rather that much satisfaction can be obtained from ordinary everyday activities that most take for granted' (Clarke and Warren 2007: 472). Where policy and the preferences of the vast majority of older people coincide is on the importance of remaining independent for as long as possible. This means that the challenge for policy-makers is to address issues that go beyond physical health and fitness. It is a welcome change that concepts such as social participation and engagement, citizenship and the 'active community' are now regularly articulated in policy documents such as *Securing Better Mental Health for Older Adults* (Philp and Appleby 2005). Likewise, the EU Green Paper *Improving the Mental Health of the Population* (EC 2005) identifies social support networks, the encourage-

ment of physical activity, and participation in community and volunteering programmes as being key factors in promoting mental health in older people.

## Social and cultural factors

Socio-economic status has a very direct influence on an individual's capacity to age
well through keeping active. 'Being lower in the social hierarchy is equivalent to more
rapid ageing' (Marmot et al. 2002, in Bowling 2005: 135). Socio-economic status
affects opportunities to participate in earlier years and determines the habits with
which individuals move towards older age, and the availability of the material
resources needed to participate in activities that promote mental well-being. A
longitudinal study in Sweden (Agahi and Parker 2005) showed that while participation rates across four categories of activity (social and cultural; physical; intellectual;
and expressive/religious) increased overall between 1992 and 2002, the rates reduced
with low education and increasing age. Interestingly, living with another person (as
opposed to living alone) was associated with higher participation rates, once again
illustrating the complex interplay between personal and social factors.

For the current generations of older people, participation in activities will, in
many cases, also be affected by gender roles. Having been brought up in a strongly
gender-differentiated world, women may be more accustomed to indoor activities
reflecting their roles in the home. Older people from different ethnic groups are also
subject to factors that may affect participation. Different cultural traditions will
influence the patterns of physical activity with which individual older people have
lived and the kinds of activities that are appropriate for them as they age. Although
much research alludes to issues of cultural and ethnic diversity, and points to cultural
factors that influence activity and participation, relatively little detailed research is
available in this area (see p. 118, 'Barriers to physical activity').

## Keeping active physically

### Physical activity and mental health

Older adults are at increased risk of physical illness which can reduce functional
activity and can be associated with high levels of psychological morbidity, particularly depression and anxiety (Katon 2003). Participation in regular physical activity
(both aerobic and strength exercises) has been shown to elicit a number of favourable
responses that contribute to healthy ageing – both indirectly and directly. For
example, physical exercise is associated with reduced blood pressure and blood fats
alongside improvements in physical function, even when started in older age. These
general health benefits will promote the vitality and confidence that sustain other
sorts of activities (e.g., social interaction) known to promote mental well-being (i.e.,
indirect effects on mental health). Physical activity is also a major modifiable risk
factor in a range of long-term conditions (LTCs). For example, abdominal obesity is

associated with cardiovascular disease, diabetes mellitus type 2 and cancer morbidity. Exercise could lessen this risk factor and consequently reduce prevalence of the physical condition and associated psychological morbidity (Schuit 2006).

Physical activity also contributes directly to intellectual, cognitive and emotional health as several studies have demonstrated. A one-year intervention programme involving exercises undertaken at home and in an exercise group resulted not only in increased muscle strength and oxygen intake and improved reaction times, but also in improved dementia-related memory function (Soya et al. 2005). In a longitudinal study in the USA, the incidence rate of dementia was significantly lower in a group of older people exercising three times a week and this corresponded to a 32 per cent reduction in risk (Larson et al. 2006). This study also cites research showing the positive effect of regular exercise for people with established Alzheimer's disease (Teri et al. 1998, and 2003, in Larson et al. 2006). It has also been shown to positively influence depression (Mather et al. 2002; Kazuhiro et al. 2006). In another study older adults were randomly allocated to a swimming pool-based aerobic exercise programme for ten weeks, while a similar, matched group had to wait to start the programme at the end of the ten-week group (the *wait-list control* group). The people in the exercise group showed increases in cognitive performance over the ten-week period whereas those in the wait-list control group did not (Hawkins et al. 1992). Although there have been few such well-designed studies, and some have demonstrated less convincing results, reviews of this literature have concluded that exercise does indeed have a positive impact upon cognition both in normal older adults and in those with early signs of Alzheimer's disease. In particular it has been found that physical exercise is beneficial for what is called **executive control** which is responsible for planning, multitasking and dealing with ambiguity (Hillman et al. 2008). It could easily be argued that such skills are relevant and important to social interactions, and hence well-being and positive mental health.

Results of cross-sectional and longitudinal studies also indicate that aerobic exercise training has anti-depressant and anxiolytic effects and protects against harmful consequences of stress (Salmon 2001). A recent randomized clinical trial of physical exercise for clinical depression has provided encouraging results (Blumenthal et al. 2007). In this study patients with major depressive disorder were assigned to one of three treatment groups: medication, exercise or a combination of both. At the end of four months the patients assigned to the exercise group alone showed as much improvement in their mood as the other two groups. Although the participants in this study were middle-aged rather than older adults there is no reason to suspect that older adults would not benefit in a similar way.

While there is now some consensus that physical activity is good for mental health there remains some uncertainty about why this should be so (Crone et al. 2005). The direct physical benefits of exercise that can be measured through blood pressure, body mass index and so on are only part of the picture. It is thought that exercise impacts upon depression by a range of mechanisms such as changing people's daily routine, increasing their interaction with others, helping them lose weight, their participation in outdoor recreation and the mastering of difficult physical and psychological challenges (Salmon 2001). In other words, exercise is probably effective by affecting the dynamic interplay between biological, psychological and social factors (Biddle and Mutrie 2001). There are several views as to how exercise may reduce anxiety. For example, it may merely provide a distraction from the causes of anxiety, or possibly the increased body temperature associated with exercise reduces muscle tension – the so-called thermogenic hypothesis (Callaghan 2004). Another hypothesis is called the Opponents Process Model which postulates that activation of physiological arousal processes in the body causes a compensatory rebound increase in relaxation (see Callaghan 2004 for a review). Whatever the physical causes of the links between exercise and reductions in anxiety, there is little doubt of its effectiveness.

## How much physical activity?

The guideline amount of physical activity needed to secure health benefits is 30 minutes a day according to the American Colleges of Sports Medicine. Until recently it was assumed that vigorous exercise is necessary, but it is now recognized that regular moderate intensity exercise delivers most of the health benefits. Such moderate intensity exercise is equivalent to walking at a rate of 3–4 mph for a healthy adult (McMurdo 2000). Although not specified, the equivalent exercise intensity for older people would probably be achieved by a somewhat slower walking rate than this.

## What kinds of physical activity?

There is an important distinction to make between 'physical activity' and 'exercise'. Many studies of the effects of physical activity on ageing focus only on leisure time 'fitness' activities. A focus on high intensity exercise has perhaps been at the expense of the sustained, lower level exercises and fitness derived from everyday life activities that are more realistic and appropriate for the functional abilities of older people (Melillo et al. 1996). The impact of retirement can be very significant, particularly for blue-collar workers, where physically demanding work may have been the norm. A recent study (Berger et al. 2005) showed a marked decrease in activity following retirement with no compensating increase in levels of activity in other areas of life to enable people to maintain recommended levels. In addition, women were shown to be far less likely to meet activity recommendations than men. The study observed that leisure time activities remained fairly constant pre- and post-retirement, suggesting that patterns set in earlier adulthood are important determinants of behaviour. The assumption that since retirement provides the time to get involved in healthy leisure pursuits, people automatically will do so, is too simplistic. In fact, in this study, not having the time to exercise was the most frequently cited deterrent.

Moreover, it has also been recognized that exercise to meet recommended levels can be taken outside formal exercise programmes. So the 30 minutes per day can be accumulated in short bouts of moderate or intense activity. Activities such as housework, gardening, climbing stairs, DIY, and so on can contribute to this target, provided the intensity equates to that of brisk walking. Gardening provides physical activity and can improve fitness and stamina, and it has been shown to have a positive effect on feelings of self-worth (Milligan et al. 2005, in Cattan 2006: 193). Interestingly in this study, the older people themselves found the main benefit of gardening to be mental stimulation – they 'felt better in themselves' (Cattan 2006: 46). They reported similar feelings in relation to other skilled, physical activities such as DIY, woodwork and upholstery, all of which gave them a sense of achievement.

There is also substantial evidence that fitness can be regained through regular physical activity, even in very old age (Fiatarone et al. 1990), and weight–bearing exercise is known to slow the rate of bone loss in older women. The benefits of exercise such as tai chi in improving balance and preventing falls is also well researched (Li et al. 2001; Xu et al. 2006).

## Where physical activity takes place

Older people also gain from the environmental and social contexts in which the physical exercise experience takes place. One study looks at two separate groups of older people, one engaged in fitness exercise, the other in dance exercise. Older people in both groups did appear to 'actively resist age' (Paulson 2005: 243), but they articulated the benefits of physical activity in quite different terms. The fitness group focused on individual health issues, cardiac measures and functional abilities, while the dance group expressed the benefits in psychological terms – the importance of ageing gracefully, 'exerting the mind over the ageing body' (Paulson 2005: 239), and the value of togetherness in the group. Similarly, the effects of exercise and music in improving mental well-being are now recognized. The combination of physical exercise and the engagement of the emotions through music appears to provide a formula for improving well-being and 'happiness' (Tilford et al. 1997). Common to these examples is the social setting in which the exercise takes place, the network and support provided in the exercise group, and the sense of purpose and belonging it gives.

For older people from ethnic minorities, the appropriate setting for physical activity is influenced by cultural factors. In a study of older British South Asians, the lack of culturally sensitive facilities meant that, for example, several women could not follow the medical advice they had received because cultural taboos about exposing their bodies to members of the opposite sex prevented them from going swimming or to a gym (Lawton et al. 2006).

*Barriers to physical activity*

Low activity levels in older people are found across the developed world. Why this is the case when the benefits have been so persuasively demonstrated has been the subject of much research. Declining physical abilities clearly play a part and are frequently cited by older people themselves. Self-perception of poor health is an important barrier to physical activity – 'my doctor told me to be careful not to over-exert myself'. A study in the USA found that the most frequently cited barrier was perceived severity of 'medical problems' (Larkin et al. 2005), specifically arthritis and cardiovascular disease, followed by, and probably linked to, lack of motivation. A study of what prevents older people from participating in leisure time physical activity found that older people mentioned a number of deterrents: physical symptoms such as painful joints and shortness of breath; fear of falling; reluctance to go out alone or in the evening; and lack of access to transport (Crombie et al. 2004).

Activity levels are also influenced by cultural expectations and norms of appropriate retirement behaviour, by low motivation and by a number of practical barriers, such as access, that older people encounter. The issue of cultural expectation and the way it may mould individual experiences is an important one. A 'lack of interest [in exercise] was by far the most powerful deterrent' (Crombie et al. 2004: 291). While acknowledging the effect, in some cases, of factors such as underlying depression, the study concluded that this was largely attributable to a set of beliefs about what are desirable levels of activity for older people, arguing that these beliefs have created attitudes and behaviours in relation to physical activity that are difficult to overcome but need to be changed (Crombie et al. 2004).

On top of this, 'fitness' is an industry that has largely been defined from the perspective of younger people. It has acquired a 'high-tech, lycra-clad' (McMurdo 2000: 1150) image focused on getting people to pursue conformity to a slim, well-muscled ideal, which can be very intimidating for middle-aged people, let alone older people. In a study of the experiences of people on exercise referral schemes, 'self-acceptance' was found to be an important measure (Crone et al. 2005). This related to body image and the recognition that physical activity is age-appropriate behaviour and that, conceived in those terms, it is achievable.

There are specific barriers affecting older people from some ethnic minority cultures. A study of older people of Pakistani or Indian origin with type 2 diabetes (Lawton et al. 2006) found that the traditional roles and norms of behaviour made it very difficult to create time for exercise. British South Asians have a strong work ethic and give priority to supporting other members of the family rather than pursuing individual interests. This means that 'taking time out for themselves to go out exercising could be interpreted as a selfish and hence a culturally inappropriate act' (Lawton et al. 2006: 47). This affected women particularly because of the cultural expectation that they would stay at home and focus on domestic responsibilities. Another study (Reijneveld et al. 2003) of Turkish immigrant communities in the Netherlands observed that cultural barriers prevented older people from exercising in front of younger women and in the vicinity of men. As a result, most participants in the study were unable to exercise at home. All these factors have implications for health promotion initiatives.

## Keeping active mentally

### Mental activity and mental health

As we have seen, research shows that keeping physically active has a positive impact on cognitive function, mood and well-being. Does keeping mentally active have similar beneficial effects? Unlike physical activity, there is no real guideline or measure for how much 'exercise' is needed to maintain mental well-being. Compared to the body of research on physical activity, there is relatively little research on the effects of intellectual activity on mental well-being. Where studies exist, they remain speculative and await further research into neurobiological and psychological processes. Published in 2001, a longitudinal analysis of leisure time activities and intellectual functioning does establish a 'rough-hewn' hypothesis (Schooler and Mulatu 2001: 479) that exposure to complex environments increases individuals' levels of intellectual functioning while exposure to simple environments decreases them. As a result, the 'intellectual benefits for middle-aged and older adults of doing intellectually challenging things in their leisure time are significant and meaningful' (Schooler and Mulatu 2001: 477). The impact of higher socio-economic status was also shown to have a positive effect. These findings echo those of studies on the relationship between complex intellectual activities and dementia or Alzheimer's disease where more research is available. One such study shows that patients with Alzheimer's disease had reduced complexity of leisure time activities at least five years before the onset of the disease (Friedland et al. 1997).

## What kinds of mental activity?

Evidence of the types of intellectual activities that are most beneficial is difficult to find. Anecdotally, activities that involve some degree of complex mental processing, such as crosswords, bridge, scrabble, sudoku, etc., are valued by older people but there is no evidence that demonstrates whether and how these activities have health benefits. That they have other benefits in terms of self-confidence seems likely. There is increasing interest in computer-based puzzles as a way of stimulating mental activity; the Alzheimer's Society cites evidence that such mental stimulation provided by, for example, Nintendo's Wii gaming console can slow the progression of the disease. A local authority in Wales has introduced this technology into residential homes for older people in a new initiative aiming to 'encourage residents to join in activities designed to keep them mobile, mentally alert, self-confident and socially interactive' (Neath Port Talbot Council 2005). Claims for this new technology may be premature but the Wii is generating support among health professionals, with doctors using it for rehabilitation (Wiihabilitation) therapy following stroke, fracture or surgery (Tanner 2008). In addition to its capacity to engross patients and offer mental stimulation, the Wii also has much physical interactivity through sports such as tennis, baseball, bowling, golf, etc. In this way, it is argued that the Wii is capable of engaging the person physically, intellectually and emotionally, and so enlivening them.

## Educational activities: life-long learning

*Older learners and public policy*

As we have seen (Chapter 3), opportunities to take part in education in later life have been linked to improvements in mental health and several theories support the role of learning and education in helping people cope with the challenges of later life as well as meeting the need for self-expression. The term 'life-long learning' is not particularly associated with older people but describes a process across the lifespan. Indeed in terms of public policy nationally and internationally, the connection between older people, ageing and education is limited. Such policy focuses mainly on the function of life-long learning in promoting 'productive roles' (Jamieson 2007), enhancing skills for work and helping people adjust to new technologies. Older people who continue to work may benefit from this 'life-long perspective' (UNESCO 1998), but in practice it tends to refer to younger people. In the UK, the policy focus has been on widening participation in education, with targets for 18–30-year-olds. Alongside this, public funding of the non-vocational and non-accredited types of extra-mural study that was popular among retired and older people in the 1970s and 1980s has ceased in the UK.

*Participants in educational activities*

An OECD study (2005) identified two key factors in relation to older people: first, that people with a history of educational attainment are more likely to participate in formal learning in older age; second, that participation declines with increasing age. In Europe, the highest levels of participation were found in Scandinavian countries. A National Adult Learning Survey in the UK (NCSR 2002) found around 64 per cent of people aged 50–59 reported some form of participation in taught learning; this figure reduced to 35 per cent for people aged 60–69 and 18 per cent for those over 70. These statistics show that a only a minority of older people engage in formal learning. A study of educational participation by older people in New Zealand found that older adults are 'typically marginalised in terms of access to education' (Findsen 2002: 5). Citing a policy discussion paper in the UK (Carlton and Soulsby 1999), Finsden concludes that 'we are likely to find that participation is strongly associated with previous educational experience, gender, race/ethnicity, and social class' (Finsden 2002: 6). In the UK, older people make up a substantial proportion of users of Adult and Community Learning provided by Local Education Authorities according to research by the Department for Education and Skills (Soule 2005), with over half of all learners on non-accredited courses being aged over 55 years. Given the withdrawal of public funding and the well-publicized cost of such study, it is likely, however, that older people on lower incomes are largely excluded.

*Motivation of older learners*

A number of studies have looked at why older people get involved in learning and study. Personal growth, acquiring new skills, and developing self-confidence have all been cited. Study as a 'mechanism to manage the transition into retirement' is identified as another incentive. Taking part in study may also relate to a quest for meaning in life as part of a process of reviewing life after retirement. Getting involved in formal or informal learning is also assumed to provide social benefits – new friends and networks. A study of older learners at Birkbeck College and the Open University in the UK (Jamieson 2007) challenges some assumptions about older people and learning. For example, social benefits were found to be much more important to younger students (Callender 1997, in Jamieson 2007), while the value of study as a source of self-confidence did not feature among older students (O'Dowd 2005), but the determination to get a qualification, even with the stress of assessment or examination, was much higher than expected – a 'drive to preserve or gain self-esteem through a socially-recognised and valued formal qualification' (Jamieson 2007: 281). This notion of achieving a meaningful identity was perceived by the older students as crucial to well-being. Further, stress-inducing events such as assessment can be stimulating and can have positive effects on the functioning and health of individuals (McEwen 2000, in Jamieson 2007).

While older people are reported as 'likely to say that learning had a positive effect on their physical, mental and emotional well-being' (Soule 2005: 91), the hard evidence linking participation in life-long learning with improvements in older people's mental health is missing; the jury is out. This may be because little research has been done rather than due to an absence of any link *per se*. However, commentators note that while many older people report an increase in self-confidence and self-esteem as a result of taking part in life-long learning, there may be others for whom the experience is far less positive. Much will depend on other factors: the quality of teaching, the environment; the attitude of staff and fellow students, etc.

*Non-formal learning: University of the 3rd Age*

The University of the 3rd Age (U3A) has perhaps filled the gap left by non-investment in non-vocational adult education courses in the UK, at least for some older learners.

Founded in France in 1972, by the early 1980s the U3A had become established in the UK and the USA. It is a self-help model of learning, with local cooperatives drawing on the knowledge and skills of their own members who 'teach' or lead informal sessions usually in members' homes. As a result, the range of subjects covered within the U3A movement is vast: art, music, comparative religion, history, philosophy and science as well as physical activities. The U3A is based on the principle of learning for pleasure. There are no accreditations, exams or assessments.

---

## Box 7.1 Life-long learning

### Case Study 1

Mrs E. is a 68-year-old woman who lives alone. She was divorced more than 30 years ago, has irregular contact with her two adult children and has no grandchildren. She has always spent a lot of time on her own and is uncomfortable in social situations. She spent her entire working life working as a technician in a research laboratory, work which she enjoyed, at which she excelled and which suited her solitary disposition. She was devastated when she had to retire and took some time to adjust. She started to attend a science group at her local University of the 3rd Age to maintain her contact with the scientific world. She also started a thorough and comprehensive compilation and review of local history records of the area in which she lives, and has a cupboard full of perfectly annotated notes and documents. One day, she says, they may be useful to the local historian or library. Right now they are a focus for personal intellectual activity, which is like a lifeline to Mrs E. She structures her life methodically, trying to have at least two or three activities a week which she says 'helps structure the empty space after retirement'.

(Unpublished research by Forte and Aitchison based on interviews conducted for the study on *Cortisol Secretory Activity* in Evans et al. 2007)

# Social activities

## Participative activities and mental health

Participation in social activities helps keep people connected and engaged with others, gives them a sense of purpose and meaning, and helps them maintain their self confidence. Many aspects of social activity are covered in other chapters (such as relationships and spirituality). Here we focus primarily on organized, participative activities. The term 'social capital' has been coined as shorthand to describe the resources available to individuals in terms of friends, family, community, etc., with each individual having a stock of 'social capital' unique to them. This may include work or work like activity such as volunteering or participation in formally organized activity as well as more informal activities. Having strong social capital is linked with high levels of social participation. Not surprisingly, social participation is also likely to result in people being more physically active and intellectually alert, pointing once again to the dynamic interplay of factors.

## What kinds of social activities?

*Day care activities*

Many activities are provided for older people and are targeted specifically at those who live alone or are isolated in the community. Some of these activities are based in purpose-built centres, while others take place in more informal settings. Public and voluntary organizations, for example, provide activities in day centres and community centres. In some cases, there have been significant improvements in recent years in the quality and variety of activities that are offered to older people. In the past, such centres have been identified with tea, biscuits and bingo – a caricature that they may still struggle to shake off. However, many now provide innovative, imaginative, challenging and stimulating activities that enable older people to enjoy themselves, interact with others and develop new skills and interests (see Table 7.1).

**Table 7.1** The Bradbury Active Age Centre, Age Concern, Kingston upon Thames

| DAY | TIME | ACTIVITY |
|---|---|---|
| Monday | 10.00–11.30 | Hypnotherapy |
| | 10.30–11.30 | The Monday Forum (topical discussion) |
| | 10.30–12.30 | Beginners' computer courses (4 weeks) |
| | 10.30–11.30 | Walking for Health – the Bradbury Weekly Walk |
| | 1.00–2.00 | Gentle exercise to music: all levels welcome |
| | 2.30–3.30 | Yoga |
| | 2.00–4.00 | Natural healing and reiki |
| | 2.00–4.00 | Scrabble |
| | | |
| Tuesday | 10.15–11.30 | Line dancing |
| | 12.00–2.30 | Indian head massage/reflexology |
| | 2.00–4.00 | Bridge/chess/board games |
| | 2.00–3.30 | Philosophy for life |
| | | |
| Wednesday | 10.30–11.30 | Weekly discussion group |
| | 10.30–12.30 | Carers' support meetings |
| | 11.15–12.15 | Bradbury Bathers (swimming group) |
| | 11.30–1.00 | Reflexology |
| | 1.15–2.45 | Art class |
| | 2.30–3.30 | French conversation |
| | | |
| Thursday | 10.30–11.30 | Keep fit |
| | 10.30–12.30 | Carers' support meetings |
| | 11.30–1.00 | My Generation – singers |
| | 10.00–1.30 | Massage treatments |
| | 2.00–3.00 | Beginners' Spanish |
| | | |
| Friday | 10.15–11.15 | Bradbury Book Club |
| | 10.00–3.30 | Massage treatments |
| | 10.30–11.30 | Basic Plus+ computer course (4 weeks) |
| | 11.30–12.30 | Computer clinic |
| | 1.00–2.00 | Bingo |
| | 2.00–3.00 | Tai chi: all levels welcome |

*Source:* (www.ageconcernkingston.org)

Despite these improvements, day centres tend to have a negative connotation. Evidence still suggests that activities are often inappropriate, and that older people use them not because they are voting with their feet but because there is nothing else available (Cattan et al. 2003). A report by the Kings Fund on day services in London (Kings Fund 2005), while acknowledging some examples of good practice, found little evidence that innovative services for older people were being developed. Further, it is very often the lonely or isolated older people who do not access these services and remain extremely hard to reach. The advent of **Healthy Living Centres** that enshrine the policy focus on physical exercise and disease prevention may have led to a sense that day centres have had their day. But for many older people, they still have a very important role as a focus for life in contact with others. There are clearly significant challenges to develop more flexible and responsive services to make them more culturally and ethnically sensitive and inclusive, and perhaps the greatest challenge of all to ensure that they are integrated into the fabric of the community and are not part-time communities that go no further than the centre door. To do this, day centres need to look outward and foster roles, activities and relationships that are integrated into people's daily lives (Clark 2001).

The Homeshare Project (Age Concern Sutton) adopts a different form of day care with weekly visits to the homes of volunteers. The scheme serves vulnerable people for whom a mainstream 'centre' is not appropriate but who need companionship. This is a versatile model for individuals who still live in the community but may be on the brink of institutional care. An evaluation of this project (Clark 2001) showed that 80 per cent of the people using the project were over 80; 50 per cent had sensory impairments and 66 per cent had restricted mobility. This is a good example of a more informal but nonetheless organized scheme that lends itself to existing communities and neighbourhoods.

*Cross-generational activities*

Research on older people living in Hong Kong showed that contact with people of different generations, in other words children and grandchildren (termed *generativity*) was the single most powerful predictor of positive well-being (Cheng et al. 2004). The role of grandparenting is considered in Chapter 6. In addition to this family role, there is much evidence of the positive impact of intergenerational relationships and activity on reported well-being among older people. There are countless projects across the UK that bring older people and young people together. Broadly, they share the same aim: to encourage older people to play an active part in the lives of children, sharing their knowledge, skills and experience, and to promote greater understanding and respect between generations. One such project is run by Age Concern Kingston upon Thames and won the Queen's Award for Community Service in 2007. It involves older volunteers working alongside children in primary schools in literacy, numeracy and science lessons. The head teacher of one of the schools has commented: 'their [older volunteers'] expertise and understanding have enriched the children's lives and a huge impact has been made on their learning, attendance at school, homework and, above all, self-esteem.' The project has recently expanded into a Learning Mentor project supporting children with the crucial transition into secondary school (see www.ageconcernkingston.org). A host of projects across the country engage the generations together to learn from one another through exchanging skills and developing supportive and stable relationships.

---

**Box 7.2** Intergenerational experiences

**Case Study 2**

Miss W. worked as a specialist tax accountant in a senior role with a leading City company. When she retired she 'began to feel a bit useless with nothing much to offer any more. Although I enjoyed my freedom from work routine and my new-found leisure activities, I felt I was simply filling the time and needed a purpose.' Five years ago she became involved in an intergenerational project helping children at a junior school with reading. Her talent for mathematics was spotted and she has supported many young children to achieve better numeracy skills. After two years with the school, she was invited to become a school governor. Her work at the school has dispelled her sense of loss following retirement and it gives her:

> a sense of job satisfaction. Sometimes my visits to school can be a little frustrating but the children are delightful and stimulating ... nothing is more rewarding than seeing a child suddenly understand. It [the Age & Youth project] is a thoroughly worthwhile project which has enhanced my retirement.
>
> (Age & Youth Project, Age Concern Kingston upon Thames.
> www.ageconcernkingston.org)

---

*Activities undertaken alone*

While there is evidence that social and cultural activities promote well-being, functioning and survival, participation in solitary activities shows less conclusive results. However, the value of such activities should not be underestimated. Presenting findings from the Growing Older Programme funded by the Economic and Social Research Council (ESRC), Bowling (2005) comments that these kinds of 'solitary-by-choice' activities were extremely important to around 48 per cent of the respondents in her study. One female participant in a recent study (Evans et al. 2007) who lives alone, enjoys the solitary days she spends pursuing her interest in scientific research. However, she recognizes that being on her own too much is not a good thing. For the majority of participants in this study, the balance between activities pursued alone and those pursued with others was important.

*Virtual social activities*

There is evidence that increasing numbers of older people are using the Internet as a tool for social networking. A recent study in Australia (Russell et al. 2008) set out to explore the relationship between Internet usage and access to social capital in later life. It found that the majority of participants made quite extensive use of the Internet to communicate with friends and family, and also to engage in wider social networks. A study in the Netherlands (Fokkema and Knipscheer 2007) evaluated an 'Internet-at-home' intervention aimed at reducing loneliness. It found that participants used email for social contact and also used the computer and Internet to pass the time. While there was a reduction in emotional loneliness, this was confined to participants with high levels of education. Other studies question the positive effects of computer and Internet use on the well-being of older people (Dickinson and Gregor 2006), suggesting that such claims may be premature. There is certainly debate (see Chapter 3) about the extent to which virtual communities can substitute for real communities in terms of connecting people and preventing loneliness and isolation.

## Work and work-like activities

*Employment*

Many older people continue in some kind of part-time paid employment or self-employment. A study of people aged 50–75 in the workforce found that the highest levels of well-being were among employed people (Roberston et al. 2004 in Walker 2005). The presence of goals set by others and the personal interactions at work, together with the status it conferred, all contributed to individuals feeling a greater level of personal control over their lives which positively influenced their sense of well-being. Huppert and Whittington (2003) also found having a job to be an important determinant of positive well-being. For some, retirement is experienced as loss. As Case Study 1 (Box 7.1) showed, having two or three things to do each week 'helps structure the empty space after retirement'. The implementation of EU legislation in relation to age discrimination has started to affect employment policies on retirement. Alongside this, changing patterns of employment, greater employment mobility and lower occupational pensions, increasing economic pressures and, in many Western European countries (especially the UK), high levels of debt mean that continuing employment beyond what is currently accepted as a normal retirement age may become more prevalent in the coming decades.

*Volunteering*

Although there is a lack of robust evidence of the mental health benefits of volunteering in older people (Windle et al. 2007), the productive nature of volunteering can have a positive effect on life satisfaction and health. Estes et al. (2003), discussing 'productive' ageing, note the shift in assumptions underpinning policy in relation to older age from a time of dependency to a new emphasis on continuing work or 'work-like' activities that help to 'maintain self independently'(Estes et al. 2003: 71). Volunteering can enable activities and roles from middle age to be maintained or replaced with new ones by transferring skills developed through one's career into new settings. Gabriel and Bowling (2004) comment on the value of the 'reciprocal' nature of volunteering. Volunteering requires commitment; it imposes an expectation on individuals that both gives structure to time and creates a mechanism for feeling valued. Recognizing the growing political and social expectations of older people engaging in volunteering, it is important to ensure that opportunities for volunteering are truly reciprocal and that volunteers are not pressurized or 're-obligated' (Erlinghagen and Hank 2006: 581).

Large numbers of older people in Europe and North America are involved in volunteering. A study in the European Union found rates of participation in volunteering were lower in Southern Europe (Spain and Italy) as compared with France, Germany and Scandinavia, and that rates increased in the 65–74 age range, typically after retirement, and declined again after 75 (Erlinghagen and Hank 2006). Rates of volunteering are also linked with socio-economic status and level of education with around 6 per cent participation among older people with little formal education and up to an average of 18 per cent among those with high levels of education. There was also a close link found between volunteering, involvement in other social activities and living in a long-term partnership. Perceived poor health was linked to low levels of volunteering. Engagement in volunteering is also influenced by the history and culture in which older people live. A long history of voluntary action and the plethora of voluntary organizations in countries like the UK present a specific context which differs from, say, Italy or Spain. Ethnic background and religious traditions also influence volunteering. For example, a study in the UK (Nazroo et al. 2004) showed that volunteering in Pakistani, Jamaican and Gujurat communities is often channelled through religion. Likewise, many white British older people participate as volunteers in support of local church activities.

## Some health promotion challenges

### Information and campaigns

Research studies note that health education campaigns in the UK have tended not to focus on older people. There is a stronger pattern of health education campaigning focused on 'seniors' in the USA (such as Senior Health Alliance Promoting Exercise (SHAPE) in Chicago and a number of examples in Hopman-Rock and Westhoff 2002). Commentators tend to agree, health promotion activities need to be framed in the context of healthy lifestyles and include incentives for older people and that this is a challenge. Identifying groups of older people at risk of inactivity and finding ways of engaging them in social and/or physical activities (Agahi and Parker 2005) is also challenging. Research into the perspectives of older people themselves underlines the need to see them as individuals for whom nuanced responses are essential. Older people need specific and personally relevant information about healthy lifestyles and about what they can do to exert control over their lives. Evidence suggests that older people are often anxious about their health and concerned that they might 'overdo it' or cause themselves harm if they increase their levels of physical activity or exercise. Information that helps them understand their physical condition and focuses on the benefits as well as the risks of exercise is important.

## Environment and access – settings for activity

Physical accessibility and the quality of the location in which organized activities take place are all vitally important. Where specialist transport provision is necessary, this can be very expensive. However, the challenge of access, as we have seen, is far wider than this. It needs to be person-centred so that initiatives really do meet the needs of the target group and are delivered in appropriate ways.

Combining health education with exercise was the focus of a major active ageing programme in the Netherlands in the 1990s (Hopman-Rock and Westhoff 2002). The programme was based on the principles of peer education and empowerment, and thus the education component was delivered by specially trained peer educators. Peer education has been shown to be 'an efficient way to transfer messages to a target group and to empower them' (Hopman-Rock and Westhoff 2002: 391). In this study participants reported very high levels of satisfaction with the programme. This was assessed against factors such as location, accessibility, size of group, duration and frequency of sessions, and atmosphere.

Whether people continue with physical activity in the long term will depend on how satisfactory the initial experience is. Health promotion focused on exercise, for example, needs to pay attention to the context (Crone et al. 2005) and the attributes of social support (staff, other users, family) that can motivate and help with adherence by older people as well as build their confidence. Regular exercise as part of everyday life in the home ideally needs to be combined with group sessions, as the effect of the social context is important (Helbostad 2004, in Cattan 2006: 192). Creating a sense of belonging through integrating opportunities for social interaction with physical exercise activities is vital.

# Role of health professionals

Health care professionals play a key role in health promotion among older people. Not only are they frequently in contact with older people, but older people themselves are most likely to approach their doctor or practice nurse for information and advice about their health and their physical activities, and are more likely to be responsive to their advice about prevention measures (Kerse et al. 2005). People with newly diagnosed diseases, for example, diabetes or another age-related chronic disease, are often receptive to the idea of making changes in their health-related behaviour, and health care professionals are in a good position to encourage an increase in physical activity as part of this behavioural shift. Studies show that the likelihood of starting new physical activities in old age, even in very old age, is very strongly linked to encouragement by health professionals to exercise (Hirvensalo et al. 2003). Similarly, in relation to social and intellectual activities, health professionals can be instrumental in encouraging older people to take part.

Recruiting older people to take part in health-promoting activity is a major challenge. The Netherlands study (Hopman-Rock and Westhoff 2002) targeted people over 65 living independently in the community with a physically inactive lifestyle.

Yet it was exactly these people that were hard to bring into the programme; most participants were already quite active. Health and care workers, for example, home care staff, are well placed to identify those who are particularly vulnerable through physically inactive lifestyles and can help steer them towards increasing their involvement in activities. However, this would also need the political commitment of senior managers in health and social care agencies in prioritizing this kind of prevention focus in the work of their frontline staff.

## Some resources

There are several resources available for older people and professionals with whom they have contact. Local organizations such as councils, libraries, Citizen's Advice Bureaux, local Age Concerns have lots of information available that is both general and locally specific. Age Concern England has an excellent series of Factsheets, regularly updated, that are available to download free of charge. For example, *Factsheet 45* – Staying healthy in later life – (Age Concern England 2008) contains good, clear information about physical activity, nutrition and other lifestyle issues written in an accessible way; *Factsheet 30* – 'leisure and learning' – (Age Concern England 2007) is also relevant.

# Conclusions

There is compelling evidence that participation in a range of types of activity (social, intellectual or physical) will improve well-being in older adults. It is often difficult to separate out which of these activities is the *active ingredient* from intervention studies that have been shown to be beneficial. For example, introduction of an exercise programme will increase physical activity but it may also extend social networks and involve intellectual engagement (such as memory and motivation). At the same time increased social participation and neighbourhood involvement may also involve more physical activity and cognitive engagement. It could be argued that it is not important to tease out the precise mechanisms by which specific activities impact upon well-being. What is important is that there is more widespread understanding of the importance of the dynamic interplay that exists between these factors, how powerful this mix is and its impact on quality of life of older adults (see Figure 7.1). More could be done to increase this awareness among the population as a whole as well as among policy-makers and service providers. Positive well-being is not only an end-product of this process but also has the power to promote motivational and cognitive characteristics in its own right. Thus, promoting positive well-being is a sustainable way of making a real impact on the lives of older adults. Increasingly people have the potential to live one-third of their lives after retirement. It is imperative to ensure those living longer are healthier as an end in itself and also in order to reduce the potential burden on the resources of health and social services, families and communities in years to come.

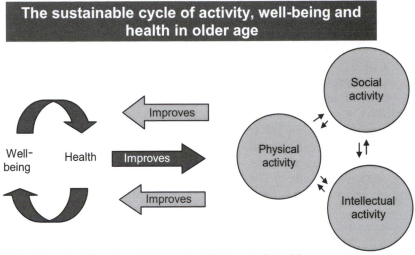

**Figure 7.1** Sustainability of activity and well-being in later life

## Reflective questions

1 What sort of policy initiatives could start to transform negative perceptions of ageing so that older generations are regarded as a rich social resource rather than an expensive drain on service provision?

2 Social activities are a key determinant in active and healthy aging. In what ways can neighbourhoods be encouraged to integrate older residents to become part of the community, for the sake of their own well-being as well as to contribute to the social capital of an area?

3 Using your own personal experience with members of your family or with clients/patients, consider what factors put individual older people at risk of inactivity.

4 What would be the key features that would ensure success in a health promotion campaign aimed at getting older people more involved in a physical activity (e.g., a walking group)?

5 Consider what steps you might take to ensure that such an exercise campaign reached older people from ethnic minority communities.

6 What factors would you need to consider in assessing the effects of an intervention on the health and well-being of individual older people?

## References

Agahi, N. and Parker, M. (2005) Are today's older people more active than their predecessors? Participation in leisure time activities in Sweden in 1992 and 2002, *Ageing & Society*, 25: 925–41.

Age Concern England (2007) Leisure and learning, *Factsheet 30*, July. Available at: www.ace.org.uk (accessed 18 Aug. 2008).

Age Concern England (2008) Staying healthy in later life, *Factsheet 45,* Nov. Available at: www.ace.org.uk (accessed 18 Aug. 2008).

Baltes, P. B. and Baltes, M. (1990) *Successful Aging: Perspectives from the Behavioural Sciences.* New York: Cambridge University Press.

Berger, U., Der, G., Mutrie, N. and Hannah, M. K. (2005) The impact of retirement on physical activity, *Ageing & Society*, 25: 181–95.

Biddle, S. J. H. and Mutrie, N. (2001) *Psychology of Physical Activity Determinants, Well-being and Interventions.* London: Routledge.

Blumenthal, J. A., Sherwood, A., Rogers, S. D. et al. (2007) Understanding prognostic benefits of exercise and antidepressant therapy for persons with depression and heart disease: the UPBEAT study. Rationale, design, and methodological issues, *Clinical Trials,* 4: 548–59.

Bowling, A. (2005) Quality of Life in Old Age. Maidenhead: Open University Press.

Bowling, A. and Gabriel, Z. (2004) An intergenerational model of quality of life in older people: comparison of analytic and lay models of quality of life, *Social Indicators Research,* 69: 1–36.

Callaghan, P. (2004) Exercise: a neglected intervention in mental health care, *Journal of Psychiatric and Mental Health Nursing,* 11: 476–83.

Cattan, M. (2006) Older people: the retirement years, in M. Cattan and S. Tilford (eds) *Mental Health Promotion.* Maidenhead: Open University Press.

Cattan, M., Newell, C., Bond, J. and White, M. (2003) Alleviating social isolation and loneliness among older people, *International Journal of Health Promotion,* 5(3): 20–30.

Cheng, S. T., Chan, A. C. M. and Phillips, D. R. (2004) Quality of life in old age: an investigation of well older persons in Hong Kong, *Journal of Community Psychology,* 32: 309–26.

Clark, C. (ed.) (2001) *Adult Day Services and Social Inclusion.* London: Jessica Kingsley.

Clarke, A. and Warren, L. (2007) Hopes, fears and expectations about the future: what do older people's stories tell us about active ageing? *Ageing & Society,* 27: 465–88.

Crombie, I. K., Irvine, L., Williams, B., McGinnis, A. R. and Peter, W. S. (2004) Why older people do not participate in leisure time physical activity: a survey of activity levels, beliefs and deterrents, *Age and Ageing,* 33(3): 287–92.

Crone, D., Smith, A. and Gough, B. (2005) 'I feel totally at one, totally alive and totally happy': a psycho-social explanation of the physical activity and mental health relationship, *Health Education Research,* 20(5): 600–11.

DH (Department of Health) (1999) *National Service Framework for Mental Health.* London: The Stationery Office.

DH (Department of Health) (2001) *National Service Framework for Older People.* London: The Stationery Office.

Dickinson, A. and Gregor, P. (2006) Computer use has no demonstrated impact on the well-being of older adults, *International Journal of Human-Computer Studies,* 64(8): 744–53.

EC (European Commission) (2005) *Improving the Mental Health of the Population: Towards a Strategy on Mental Health for the European Union.* Brussels: Health and Consumer Protection Directorate.

Erlinghagen, M. and Hank, K. (2006) The participation of older Europeans in volunteer work, *Ageing & Society*, 26: 567–84.

Estes, C., Biggs, A. and Phillipson, C. (2003) *Social Theory and Social Policy on Ageing*. Buckingham: Open University Press.

Evans, P., Forte, D., Jacobs, C. et al. (2007) Cortisol secretory activity in older people in relation to positive and negative well-being, *Psychoneuroendocrinology*, 32: 922–30.

Fiatarone, M. A., Marks, E. C., Ryan, N. D., Lipsitz, L. A. and Evans, W. J. (1990) High-intensity strength training in nonagenarians: effects on skeletal muscle, *Journal of the American Medical Association*, 263: 3029–34.

Findsen, B. (2002) *Older Adults and Learning: A Critique of Participation and Provision*. Available at: www.life-longlearning.cqu.edu.au/2002/papers/Findsen.pdf (accessed 24 May 2008).

Fokkema, T. and Knipscheer, K. (2007) Escape loneliness by going digital: quantitative and qualitative evaluation of a Dutch experiment in using ICT to overcome loneliness among older adults, *Aging & Mental Health*, 11(5): 496–504.

Friedland, R. P., Smyth, K., Esteban-Santillan, C. et al. (1997) Premorbid environmental complexity is reduced in patients with Alzheimer's disease (AD) as compared to age and sex matched controls: results of a case-control study, in K. Iqbal, B. Winblad and H. Wisniewski (eds) *Neurobiology of Aging*. New York: Wiley.

Gabriel, E. and Bowling, A. (2004) Quality of life in old age from the perspectives of older people, in A. Walker and C. Hagan Hennessey (eds) *Growing Older: Quality of Life in Old Age*. Maidenhead: Open University Press.

Glass, T. A., de Leon, C. M., Marottoli, R. A. and Berkman, L. F. (1999) Population-based study of social and productive activities as predictors of survival among elderly Americans, *British Medical Journal*, 319: 478–83.

Havighurst, R. (1963) Successful aging, in R. Williams, C. Tibbit and W. Donahue (eds) *Processes of Aging*. New York: Atherton pp. 299–320.

Hawkins, H. L., Kramer, A. F. and Capaldi, D. (1992) Aging, exercise and attention. *Psychology and Aging*, 7: 643–53.

Hillman, C. H., Erickson, K. I. and Kramer, A. F. (2008) Be smart, exercise your heart: exercise effects on brain and cognition, *Nature Reviews Neuroscience*, 9: 58–65.

Hirvensalo, M., Heikkinen, E., Lintumen, T. and Rantanen, T. (2003) The effect of advice by health care professionals on increasing physical activity of older people, *Scandinavian Journal of Medicine and Science in Sports*, 13: 231–6.

Hopman-Rock, M. and Westhoff, M. H. (2002) Dissemination and implementation of 'Aging Well and Healthily': a health-education and exercise programme for older adults, *Journal of Aging and Physical Activity*, 10: 382–95.

Huppert, F. A. and Whittington, J. E. (2003) Evidence for the independence of positive and negative well-being: implications for quality of life assessment, *British Journal of Health Psychology*, 8(1): 107–22.

Jamieson, A. (2007) Higher education study in later life: what is the point? *Ageing & Society*, 27: 363–84.

Katon, W. (2003) Clinical and health services relationships between major depression, depressive symptoms, and general medical illness, *Biological Psychiatry*, 54: 216–26.

Kazuhiro, Y., Nakahara, R., Kumano, H. and Kuboki, T. (2006) Yearlong physical activity and depressive symptoms in older Japanese adults: cross-sectional data from the Nakanojo Study, *The American Journal of Geriatric Psychiatry*, 14(7): 621–3.

Kerse, N., Elley, C. R., Robinson, E. and Arroll, B. (2005) Is physical activity counseling effective for older people? A cluster randomized controlled trial in primary care, *Journal of the American Geriatric Society*, 53: 1951–6.

Kings Fund (2005) *The Business of Caring: Kings Fund Enquiry into Care Services for Older People in London*. London: Kings Fund.

Larkin, J. M., Black, D. R., Blue, C. and Templin, T. (2005) Perceived barriers to exercise in people 65 and older: recruitment and population campaign strategies, *American College of Sports Medicine*, 37(5): S12.

Larson, E. B., Wang, L., Bowen, J. D. et al. (2006) Exercise is associated with reduced risk for incident dementia among persons 65 years of age and older, *Annals of Internal Medicine* (American College of Physicians), 144(2): 73–81.

Lawton, J., Ahmad, N., Hanna, L., Douglas, M. and Hallowell, N. (2006) 'I can't do any serious exercise': barriers to physical activity among people of Pakistani and Indian origin with Type 2 diabetes, *Health Education Research*, 21(1): 43–54.

Li, J., Hong, Y. and Chan, K. (2001) Tai chi: physiological characteristics and beneficial effects on health, *British Journal of Sports Medicine*, 35(3): 148–56.

Mather, A. S., Rodriguez, C., Guthrie, M. F. et al. (2002) A randomised controlled trial of the effects of exercise on depressive symptoms in older people with depression, *Age and Ageing*, 31 (S1): 39.

McMurdo, M. (2000) A healthy old age: realistic or futile goal? *British Medical Journal*, 321(7269): 1149–51.

Melillo, K. D., Futrell, M., Williamson, E. et al. (1996) Perceptions of physical fitness and exercise among older adults, *Journal of Advanced Nursing*, 23(3): 542–7.

Nazroo, J., Bajekal, M., Blane, D. and Grewal, I. (2004) Ethnic inequalities, in A. Walker and C. Hagan Hennessy (eds), *Growing Older: Quality of Life in Old Age*. Maidenhead: Open University Press.

NCSR (National Centre for Social Research) (2002) *National Adult Learning Survey*. London: NCSR and Department for Education and Skills.

Neath and Port Talbot Council (2005) *Wii Are Never Too Old for New Technology*. Available at: www.neath-porttalbot.gov.uk/pressreleases (accessed 23 May 2008).

Nimrod, G. and Adoni, H. (2006) Leisure styles and life satisfaction among recent retirees in Israel, *Ageing & Society*, 26: 607–30.

O'Dowd, M. (2005) Learning from childhood to mature adulthood: what makes people want to learn to learn and keep on learning, *Compare*, 35(3): 321–38.

OECD (Organisation for Economic Co-operation and Development) (2005) *Promoting Adult Learning*. Paris: OECD.

Paulson, S. (2005) How various 'cultures of fitness' shape subjective experiences of growing older, *Ageing & Society*, 25: 229–44.

Philp, I., and Appleby, L. (2005) *Securing Better Mental Health for Older Adults*. London: The Stationery Office.

Reijneveld, S. A., Westhoff, M. and Hopman-Rock, M. (2003) Promotion of health and physical activity improves the mental health of elderly immigrants: results of a group randomised controlled trial among Turkish immigrants in the Netherlands aged 45 and over, *Journal of Epidemiology and Community Health*, 57(6): 405–11.

Rowe, J. and Kahn, R. (2000) Successful aging and disease prevention, *Advances in Renal Replacement Therapy*, 7: 70–7.

Russell, C., Campbell, A. and Hughes, I. (2008) Ageing, social capital and the Internet: findings from an exploratory study of Australian silver surfers, *Australasian Journal on Ageing*, 27(20): 78–82.

Salmon, P. (2001) Effects of physical exercise on anxiety, depression, and sensitivity to stress: a unifying theory, *Clinical Psychology Review*, 21: 33–61.

Schooler, C. and Mulatu, M. S. (2001) The reciprocal effects of leisure time activities and intellectual functioning in older people: a longitudinal analysis, *American Psychological Association*, 16(3): 466–82.

Schuit, A. J. (2006) Physical activity, body composition and healthy ageing, *Science and Sports*, 21: 209–13.

Scottish Executive (2003) *National Programme for Improving Mental Health and Well-being: Action Plan 2003–06*. Edinburgh: Scottish Executive.

Soule, A. (2005) Lifestyles and leisure interests, in Department for Work and Pensions, *Focus on Older People*. London: The Stationery Office.

Soya, H., Kato, M., Sakamaki, Y., Motoyama, T. and Asada, T. (2005) Enhanced memory function of elderly people by mild intensity exercise intervention: Tone Project, *Psychogeriatrics*, 5(4): A74–5.

Tanner, L. (2008) Doctors use Wii games for rehab therapy. New York Associated Press. Available at: www.news.findlaw.com (accessed 24 May 2008).

Tilford, S., Delaney, F. and Vogels, M. (1997) *Effectiveness of Mental Health Interventions: A Review*. London: Health Education Authority.

UNESCO (United Nations Educational, Scientific and Cultural Organization) (1998) *World Declaration on Higher Education for the Twenty-First Century: Vision and Action*. Paris: UNESCO.

Walker, A. and Hennessey, C. H. (eds) (2004) *Growing Older: Quality of Life in Old Age*. Maidenhead: Open University Press.

Walker, A. and Hagan Hennessey, C. (eds) (2005) *Growing Older: Understanding Quality of Life in Old Age*. Maidenhead: Open University Press.

WHO (World Health Organisation) (2002) *Active Ageing: A Policy Framework*. Geneva: WHO.

Windle, G., Hughes, D., Linck, P. et al. (2007) *Public Health Interventions to Promote Mental Well-being in People Aged 65 and Over: Systematic Review of Effectiveness and Cost-effectiveness. NICE Evidence Reviews*. Bangor: University of Wales.

Xu, D., Li, J. and Hong, Y. (2006) Effects of long-term Tai Chi practice and jogging exercise on muscle strength and endurance in older people, *British Journal of Sports Medicine*, 40(1): 50–4.

# 8 Coping, choice and control: pathways to positive psychological functioning and independence in later life
## Maureen Mickus and Tom Owen

## Editor's foreword

This final chapter, based on older people's priorities for mental health and well-being, focuses on the importance of retaining independence and control in later life. The chapter starts by reviewing some of the theoretical concepts relating to coping, including issues around spirituality. Barriers to independence, choice and control are considered from a wide range of perspectives, including mobility, ageism, frailty and long-term care, end of life issues, and how services approach them. Importantly, the chapter gives the reader a framework on which to build realistic and evidence-based interventions to support older people's coping strategies, independence and control.

## Introduction

Retaining maximum independence with a good quality of life is a primary goal in later life. Independence is a deeply embedded value of those Westernized cultures with an individualist orientation. A focus on interdependence and community may play equally salient roles in collectivist cultures, where individual needs take less precedence (Wray 2004). Research has extensively documented the many factors that limit independence among older persons, including those that are not easily modifiable such as chronic illnesses or disabilities. Independence is also influenced by environmental factors, including living arrangements, and broader macro-level forces, such as public policies related to home and community-based care or poverty.

The purpose of this chapter is to highlight key factors that affect the ability of individuals to retain independence in later life, with a focus on those related to psychological functioning across various settings. Effective coping strategies, choice and control in particular are associated with high psychological well-being and are helpful for an older person wishing to remain independent for as long as possible. These concepts are also linked to a growing interest in 'successful ageing' (Rowe and

Kahn 1998; Depp and Jeste 2006) for which high psychological or cognitive functioning is essential. Interest in successful ageing approaches for maintaining independence suggests the development of more inclusive models of psychological functioning in later life, with emphasis not just on psychopathology, but also on positive psychological states (Fernandez-Ballesteros 2006). Understanding the attributes and conditions that are linked to psychological well-being is relevant to how older adults manage in the face of multiple losses and disease.

## Independence

Older people are not a homogeneous group with the same needs and circumstances. Contrary to typical Western stereotypes, many older people are living healthy, active and independent lives. Research tells us that typically people in older age feel 25 years younger than their age, and nearly three-quarters of people aged between 65 and 69 years rate their life as 'so good it could not be better' or 'very good', compared with between a half and a third of those in older age groups (Bowling et al. 2002). While this does not reflect the global picture of ageing, it does illustrate the general trend in Western countries of a more active older age group. Yet despite this, older adults are often viewed as passive consumers of health and welfare services rather than as citizens whose contribution as unpaid carers, volunteers and community members goes unrecognized. The World Health Organization's policy report (WHO 2002) calls for a shift in attitudes to older people towards an 'active ageing' agenda, where there is emphasis on national policies which support social inclusion among older people. The recent WHO (2007) initiative on age-friendly cities, which examined key factors in promoting inclusion and accessibility for older people within communities, also reflects this stance. Most importantly, this agenda for active ageing reflects the priorities of older people themselves. Older people have prioritized individually tailored services which support independence and the provision of information, advice, preventative services are considered crucial in meeting this priority (JRF 2004a).

Barriers within the social environment, poverty, poor health status and reduced social networks are just a few of the key factors that continue to restrict independence and inclusion of older people (Scharf et al. 2002). There is also some concern that the active ageing agenda, while positive for those who remain physically and mentally fit, has less meaning to those who are struggling with disability and are at risk of not receiving the support they need simply to manage their daily lives.

## Coping strategies

Living with a chronic illness is commonplace in later life. Nearly 80 per cent of older adults have at least one chronic disease and 50 per cent have at least two (CDCP 2003). These rates represent extensive disability, functional loss and often pain. In addition, ageing is often accompanied by social and occupational losses. For example, death of a partner and/or friends are considered normative events, but can still be highly devastating to older persons, leading to social isolation or depression. The ability of an individual to cope with the many changes in later life is critical for maintaining independence, although coping styles vary widely. Coping is understood as 'constantly changing cognitive and behavioural efforts to manage specific external and/or internal demands that are appraised as taxing or exceeding the resources of the person' (Lazarus and Folkman 1984: 14). Individuals use various styles to respond to stressful situations. One of the most frequently cited theories in the stress literature originated from Lazarus and Folkman (1984) who contended that either emotion-focused or problem-focused coping styles would contribute towards resolving a stressful situation, and thereby lead to a positive psychological state. Conversely, efforts that do not lead to resolution of the stressor could result in distress.

Problem-focused strategies may include planful problem-solving, confronting, managing or changing the stressor. These approaches typically are used when the problem seems alterable. Emotion-focused strategies may include escape avoidance, wishful thinking, seeking social support, trying to feel better about the stressor and downward comparisons. An individual is more likely to utilize emotion-focused coping in cases where the problem is perceived as out of one's control, such as a terminal illness. Similarly, Almberg et al.'s (1997) study of older caregivers found that emotion-focused coping was used by those at risk for burnout as compared to problem-focused coping for those not at risk. These findings also indicated that female caregivers were more likely than males to use emotion-focused approaches.

The concept of emotion-focused and problem-focused coping has been more recently revised as Folkman and Greer (2000) proposed a model based on meaning-based coping. Meaning-based coping allows the individual to experience positive psychological functioning, even if stress has not been resolved. This new model allows for both positive and negative emotions to co-exist during periods of extreme stress. It may result in the development of new goals, positive re-appraisal, or spiritual beliefs that allow an individual to experience positive psychological well-being in the midst of negative stressors. Blanchard-Field et al. (1995) conducted research with both young and older adults and found that older adults were more likely to be proactive or problem-focused in solving everyday instrumental problems, but more likely to use avoidant-denial strategies for interpersonal problems as compared with young adults. The authors concluded that older people were more effective in solving everyday problems overall, suggesting a maturation advantage, where experience in trying out various coping strategies over many years results in more effective solutions.

Despite the advantage of experience in coping with adversity, older adults are still likely to struggle with what Godfrey and Tenby (2004) refer to as 'daily hassles', everyday problems that can readily impact on mental well-being. The combination of sensory loss, arthritis, pain, lack of mobility, cognitive changes and reduced support systems have the potential for even simple tasks to become a serious challenge and a reminder of one's own frailty. The accumulation of problems relating to managing the home, getting out and about, difficulties in simply opening a jar or picking up something that has dropped on the floor can lead to low self-esteem and depression.

Spiritual or religious beliefs serve as a key coping mechanism for many older adults with daily hassles or more long-term stressors. In general, older adults tend to rate religion and spirituality as a more central source of strength than other age groups (McFadden 1995), and several longitudinal studies have demonstrated that the importance of religion decreased during young and middle ages, but grew considerably in later life (Wink and Dillon 2001). Disagreement exists on whether religiousness increases with age. Rather than concluding that individuals become increasingly religious with age, a cohort effect offers a more likely explanation (Davie and Vincent 1998). The current population of elders grew up in a period where religion played a more prominent role in their lives than today's young and middle-aged adults, whose perspectives towards religion may not change in old age.

Both religion and spirituality, however, can provide an important buffer for many older adults helping them to manage stress. Koenig et al. (2001) reviewed over 850 studies, the majority of which involved older adults with chronic illnesses or disabilities, and cited a definitive link between religious involvement and greater life satisfaction, lowered levels of depression and anxiety, and greater hope and optimism. Similarly, in a large survey in the USA on the role of religion and coping, Krause (2002) found that older persons who feel closer to God are more likely to be optimistic, and tended to report higher levels of psychological well-being. Cultural variations should be noted, however, as ethnic minorities, for example, older African Americans, tended to obtain greater health benefits from religious involvement as compared to non-Hispanic white Americans.

Another effective mechanism for managing stress is based on social comparison theory which suggests that people compare themselves to others to evaluate or cope with their own condition (Festinger 1954). Wills (1981) proposed two types of comparisons. When individuals feel threatened or perceive a stressor to be unalterable, they are like to make downward comparisons to feel better or improve self-esteem, for example: 'I'm not in as bad of shape as she is.' Upward comparisons may be a source of encouragement or inspiration, for example: 'He has managed to remain active with his condition, then I can too.' However, some authors have suggested that both upward and downward comparisons may be detrimental. Downward comparisons may be an uncomfortable reminder of future deterioration and upward comparisons unpleasant reminders that others are better off (Frieswijk et al. 2004). Furthermore, in a qualitative study of individuals with serious disabilities and chronic illnesses, Dewar (2003) found that downward comparisons made by others, namely health professionals, had a deleterious effect on the individual. When the physician suggested to their patient that they were not as badly off as some of the physician's other patients with cancer, the patient felt as if their circumstances were minimized and that the comments suggested they were not coping well. Nonetheless, this study provided overall support for the role of social comparisons when made by the individual, or what Dewar deemed 'boosting' in an effort to cope with serious health challenges.

One of the most promising theories for coping in later life is known as Selective Optimization with Compensation (Baltes and Baltes 1990). People select domains that are important to them, optimizing resources for success and compensating for losses. *Selection* is based on the concept that older adults have a reduced capacity and loss of functioning that requires a reduction in performance in most life domains. As a result, the individual may reprioritize goals that are better suited to their functional level. *Optimization* suggests that it is possible to maintain performance in some areas through continued practice and the use of new technologies, as it relates to maximizing performance of the individual. *Compensation* becomes relevant when life tasks require a level of capacity beyond the current level of the older adult's performance potential. This necessitates adapting to current or anticipated limitations. These strategies have been shown to be helpful in many ways, including as a buffering effect when an older adult is faced with restricted personal resources, such as lowered socio-economic status (Jopp and Smith 2006).

Similar to Selective Optimization with Compensation, emphasis on prioritizing goals according to energy or functional levels, socio-emotional selectivity theory predicts that, as perceived time left diminishes, people discard peripheral relationships and focus on important ones, such as those with close family members and friends (Carstensen 1992). This approach suggests that older adults do not simply react to social networks but rather take an active stance in managing these. Despite an overall decline in the number of relationships, this process appears to be positively related to affective well-being in older adults, and may even promote it by enabling them to focus their limited time and energy on relationships that are most beneficial, while avoiding those that are inconsequential or stressful. A growing body of research exists to support both Selective Optimization with Compensation and socio-emotional selectivity theories, both appearing to be broadly generalizable (Burnett-Wolle and Godbey 2007).

Many approaches used by older adults for coping seem readily categorized as adaptive or maladaptive. However, some strategies such as denial or avoidance behaviour, while generally viewed as maladaptive, may be necessary in the short term as an individual adjusts to a new situation. Similarly, use of humour is typically viewed as an effective approach for coping, but may be maladaptive if it prevents the individual from taking important steps to resolve the stressor where more active-oriented behaviour is needed. Understanding the specific context of the stressor, such as adjusting to a new situation (for example, loss of driving) is only one factor in determining which coping style will be used, whereas a much broader range of factors are likely to be involved, such as education, gender, ethnicity, personality, motivation and health status.

To what degree do stress and associated coping hamper an older individual's overall psychological functioning, self-care behaviour and level of independence? In the short term, stress may actually lead to positive outcomes, including motivating a person to adopt healthier behaviours. Chronic stress and lack of effective coping, however, have been repeatedly documented as harmful, both physically and psychologically, and thus subsequently exert an adverse effect on the individual's ability to retain maximum independence.

---

**Box 8.1** Independence and control

**Case study 1**

Edna Thompson is an 84-year-old female whose husband died suddenly last year. Their marriage lasted 53 years and during that time, Mr Thompson had sole responsibility for the financial management of the household (e.g., paying bills) which is now a task that Edna has taken over, but with some difficulty. Edna raised three children and never worked outside the home. Her physical health is fair, but she is greatly concerned about her failing eyesight with the onset of macular degeneration. She lives alone in a one-storey home and no longer drives. Several of her children are worried about their mother's ability to live independently, but Edna has firmly stated that she wants to remain in her own home. She discusses the situation with her friends from church and often remarks, 'At least I am in my own home and not in the nursing facility where other people I know had to go'.

Mrs Thompson faces a number of threats to her cherished independence including financial security, possible decline in functional performance due to failing eyesight and the added stressor related to managing on her own as a widow. She takes pride in her ability to remain in her own home, but is likely to require assistance with day-to-day activities from friends and family in the future. Formal care providers may need to be involved. Having a support system of friends, adult children and the availability of a formal network of carers can be critical in helping an individual remain in the setting of their choice.

---

## Choice and control with increasing frailty

Older people are often highly skilled in adapting to and compensating for disability (Reed et al. 2003), but this can be more problematic for those older people who experience high levels of frailty that threaten their independence. Although one's level of disability or dependency is relevant, an individual's *perceived* sense of autonomy is paramount in determining one's quality of life. In other words, an older adult in poor health who retains control over decisions, including the assistance received, may still view their situation positively. Older persons with little perceived sense of control in their lives are likely to feel helpless and believe their coping to be unsuccessful (Gignac et al. 2000). Margaret describes how her life as a frail older person had turned into a struggle simply to exist:

> I have become acutely aware of the fact that my life has disintegrated into two distinct parts. There is the one that I have always regarded as the real me, the outgoing sociable person with a wide range of interests and contacts. The other is the part of my life that is responsible for the management of my

daily personal affairs. Recently, however, I have realised that I can no longer manage this juggling act. The onward creep of physical decrepitude has become more and more demanding. My needs are more varied – so much so that it almost takes on an existence of its own.

(Owen 2005: 26)

Many older people in Margaret's position experience multiple co-existing health conditions which, coupled with sensory, physical and/or mental impairment, may require the attention of a range of health and care professionals. Older people can often experience what is described as the 'revolving door syndrome' (Cartier 2003), whereby life is characterized by endless admissions to hospital and visits from professionals in response to the various health complaints that they experience. Attending appointments, arranging support and transport, waiting for referrals, completing assessments and managing care packages can be both exhausting and highly debilitating for those with limited energy and capacity. One's existence becomes associated with uncontrollable health problems rather than with the positive aspects of life.

Maintaining control in long-term care settings, such as institutions, or care homes, can be extremely challenging. Older people living in long-term care settings have substantial and complex health care needs. In 2006, a comprehensive survey of UK care home residents identified that over two-thirds of older people in care homes had neurodegenerative disease such as dementia, a stroke or Parkinson's disease. It is estimated that up to 82 per cent of residents experience 'confusion', 'memory-loss', 'depression' or 'agitation' (Bowman et al. 2004; BUPA Care Homes 2006). While there is evidence of good practice within some care homes in promoting well-being among such residents, a common experience in these settings leaves many older people socially isolated, and deprived of self-esteem, social stimulation and lacking – as older people describe it, 'personhood'. Critics have compared many of these outcomes in care homes to Goffman's (1961) observations of insane asylums several decades ago in which choice and control were severely compromised.

There are systemic factors that impact upon choice and control in long-term care. Structured inflexible routines, lack of resources, lack of training can all be a barrier to a positive culture where older people retain control of their lives (Owen and NCHRDF 2006). In addition, facilities may place a higher premium on safety and less on the need for individual autonomy or control. The extent to which residents are able to exercise choice and control relates most directly to the quality of relationships that older people in long-term care have with staff (Brown-Wilson, forthcoming PhD). A positive culture which supports staff in engaging with older people at a personal level, and that recognizes the importance of reciprocity, is important for supporting choice and control. A less restrictive culture of care is emerging, including homes where even individuals with severe mental frailty are being engaged in making decisions about both their own personal lives and the structures and routines of the setting. Examples of these new models include Milford care homes in the UK in which staff support residents by actively engaging them in decision-making, particularly those who are withdrawn or have communication difficulties (www.milfordcare.co.uk). In the USA, Eden Alternative homes recognize helplessness as one of the key plagues for residents and strive to return control to their lives and to the facility staff (www.edenalt.org).

## Societal impact

Even if older people have developed successful strategies to cope or retain control over decisions, larger social influences may threaten their feelings of independence, control and self-worth. In Western cultures, a pervasive view of older adults is one of *vulnerability*, and these societal attitudes and behaviours may be so deeply rooted so that they can be very difficult to recognize and even harder to challenge. 'Elderly' or 'old age' confers negative connotations, inferring weakness, incapacity, and a lack of sexuality or attractiveness. The media, among other sources, conveys messages that older people are passive, vulnerable and a burden to society rather than an asset. Policy-makers often overlook the needs of elders (Riseborough 2000). In general, older persons are portrayed as 'slowing down', 'stupid' or 'dependent', and as a result the views of older people are not heard or valued (Seymour et al. 2005). Collectively, these images may become self-fulfilling prophecies for older individuals and seriously undermine their sense of control, independence and well-being.

Bytheway et al. (2007) describe how our behaviour toward older people is influenced by broader cultural stereotypes. It is not uncommon to assume an older person is incapacitated, unless there is evidence to suppose otherwise. These authors describe how older people may experience 'infantilization', where practitioners adopt 'elder speak' – a higher pitch condescending tone, which reinforces the sense of vulnerability experienced by older people. While families may provide a very supportive role to older people, they too can inadvertently take control over decision-making for their relative, perceiving it to be in the best interests of the older person themselves. This, however, does not negate the pressures on the older carer. There is evidence which shows that depression and anxiety are common among people who become informal carers (SPRU 2001; Doran et al. 2003), added to which, a substantial number of carers are themselves permanently sick or disabled (National Statistics 2004). Caring can therefore seriously affect older carers' physical and mental health (Box 8.2).

---

**Box 8.2.** Caring and older people: two case studies

The 2001 Census revealed that over 1.5 million men and women aged 60 or over provide unpaid care in the UK (Buckner and Yeandle 2005). Being a carer in older age can be a challenging experience, as older carers provide care while they may be in need of help for themselves because of the consequences of ageing. The following case studies represent some of the experiences that different older carers face in their everyday life.

### Case study 1

Irene is a 75-year-old widow who lives with Thomas, her adult son with learning disabilities. Irene finds it more and more difficult to run some household chores, such as lifting the washing or turning the mattress, and she doesn't have any help with these from Thomas. Thomas cannot be left alone at any time as he is not aware of danger, and this has a major impact on Irene's ability to socialize. Irene's major worry is that if she falls very sick sometime, Thomas won't be able to call for help.

### Case study 2

Carl is 72-year-old and cares for his wife, Theresa, who has a long-term disabling illness. Carl recently had a hip replacement, but he still lifts Theresa in and out of bed. Carl asked and obtained some assistance for Theresa through social services, but he struggled to pay the amount he was charged for that. Also, Theresa felt uncomfortable to be moved in and out of bed by the nurses, as they were strangers for her. As a result, Carl decided to quit the help from social services. His only source of help now is Sue, a life-long friend of Theresa, who he calls every time he can't manage on his own. Sue, however, has her own health problems too.

Consider what short-, medium- and long-term mental health promotion interventions could provide support for Irene and Carl.

## Control and coping at the end of life

Little is known from research about older people's experience of the last year of their life, however, there is general consensus that a good death involves privacy, dignity, good quality care in comfortable surroundings, with adequate pain relief and appropriate support in keeping with their preferences (GMC 2002). The evidence suggests that older people at the end of life can experience particularly poor quality of life with limited choice, control and independence. For many the last months and years of life involve 'living on thin ice' (Lynn and Adamson 2003) with general, non-specific deterioration in health and quality of life with periods of acute illness. Older adults with deteriorating health are likely to face repeated hospital admissions, under–recognition or control of symptoms, lack of preventive planning and inadequate home support. Seymour et al.'s (2005) literature review of end of life care demonstrated that the needs of older people are often not prioritized to the same extent as those of younger people with the same level of need and, in particular, they are less likely to die in their preferred place of care. Many die in hospital on busy wards, which are not conducive to privacy, personal communication and control for patients and their family members.

Every older person will have a different way of coping with the realization that they are approaching 'finitude', and their readiness to talk about death and dying may alter as their own circumstances change. For some older people, death may provide a release from chronic pain, it may be communicated as something that the older person is ready to accept. Others may find that it is too painful to think about. As noted earlier, humour can be a useful coping mechanism and is often used in acknowledging that death may be around the corner. Some older people will focus on the practical aspects of dying such as funeral arrangements or dealing with personal affairs. Finding meaning, or spirituality, can also be important for older people as they approach the end of life (MacKinlay 2005). For others, there can be a real wish to express the fact that they are dying, and to talk about their fears, their hopes and their wishes for what they would like to happen as they reach the final stage of life. In a study of quality of life among 75-year-olds, Howarth (1998) noted that in 58 per cent of the interviews, the issue of death was raised without being prompted.

Exerting a sense of control, talking about death and communicating one's wishes can be important for an individual near the end of life, although others may be uncomfortable with these discussions. Similarly, health professionals often struggle to respond to questions about death and dying, ignoring an older person's wish to openly discuss dying, diverting attention to safer areas of conversation (Albinsson and Strang 2002; Hopkinson and Hallett 2002). A survey by Help the Aged (2006) demonstrated that practitioners feel that they have neither the time nor the skills or training to support older people who are dying. Choice and control at the end of life may be particularly thwarted in long-term care settings, as evidenced by the following quote from a resident: 'Death is such a taboo subject. It's a big problem because all of us are so near to death. By 90 you can't get much nearer without knowing that it is around the corner, and we need to be able to express that sometimes if we want to' (Owen and NCHRDF 2006: 26).

Without sufficient and accurate information, older adults may be unaware of what end of life care choices are available, unable to challenge decisions made on their behalf or to prevent their choices from being undermined (Clarke et al. 2006). While advance planning for end of life care is generally ideal, there is a considerable confusion over when decisions should be made or even over what constitutes the end of life stage.

## Impact of formal service provision

Formal or paid services can play an essential role in supporting the independence of older adults in the face of declining health. A wide range of services such as assistance with activities of daily living such as bathing, dressing, meal preparation and supportive housing or social services may be available in communities, although individuals may be reluctant to accept help. Accepting services or assistance is often inconsistent with one's self-image as an independent adult, and may represent an admission of weakness or failure. There may be an unwillingness to acknowledge certain types of need, whether to oneself or to someone else (Howse 2002). Maintaining one's identity and sense of control, which have been built up over a lifetime can be more important than accepting formal services (Baldock and Hadlow 2002).

Older people may have negative images of services and low expectations of the benefits they deliver. Service users are sometimes viewed as people who are confused, without a caring family, who can no longer decide for themselves and are too poor to pay for themselves. Some older people associate use of services as a class issue, and perceive that they would have nothing in common with the people who use services. For others some services are viewed as too expensive to be an option (Baldock and Hadlow 2002). In addition, there could be moral or cultural conflicts involved in service usage. Older adults may believe that assistance should be provided exclusively by family members, and that assistance from formal providers represents a failure within the family system. Elders may have no problem acknowledging their need for assistance, but their preference or insistence that help is given by someone whom they trust and have a close pre-existing relationship, such as family or friends, may lead to formal services being blocked, even when it is questionable whether the older person's needs are being met by family care (Howse 2002).

Older people who have been socially isolated for a long period of time may need additional time to build trust and relationships with new people who are offering assistance. Attending a social or community group for the first time can be frightening and intimidating, and may add to stress rather than alleviate it (Cattan 2002). Community and day centres are viewed negatively by some older people as they feel 'fussed over' and 'patronized'. Activities may be considered too generic and not tailored to suit individual needs, and may not provide older people with the opportunity to learn or share skills. Many older people dislike sitting in large groups with people with whom they have nothing in common. These groups may also be too noisy for people with hearing difficulties.

## Older people in prison

Of course not all older people are living in the community. Older people in prison, for example, face many of the issues mentioned above: stigma, isolation, loneliness and fear of dying alone. However, prisons are not geared for the growing number of older prisoners, which is starting to be acknowledged and addressed by agencies such as Age Concern, Restore50Plus, the Prison Reform Trust and others (Prison Reform Trust 2006). Consider the following case studies in Box 8.3.

---

**Box 8.3** Imprisonment and older people: two case studies

Older people form one of the fastest growing sub-sections of the prison population. This trend is set to continue as a result of policy change in relation to sentencing laws, and more generally in increases in people's life expectancy. The following short case studies represent some of the experiences older people face while imprisoned.

### Case study 1

Brian was an older person entering the prison system for the first time later in life. Brian felt shocked, anxious and stressed in adjusting to a new environment and found being separated from his family difficult. He became socially isolated from other inmates and was generally portrayed as a 'loner', with limited social support networks. He felt vulnerable and at risk of violence from other prisoners and feared the possibility of dying while in prison.

**Case study 2**

Jim, on the other hand, was an inmate who had grown old in the prison system. Having spent many years institutionalized, Jim was familiar with the rules and regime of the prison and therefore got on well with other inmates and staff. However, Jim's mobility in the prison was becoming increasingly restricted. He was unable to participate in work or physical activity, which was important in alleviating the monotony and stress of prison life.

## The physical environment

For many older people, 'maintaining a home' has always been the main source of choice and control. Home is an essential aspect of one's identity, although for those individuals struggling to maintain physical and mental health, upkeep of the home can be a challenge. One might find that the home no longer reflects a positive identity; it may be unkempt or poorly maintained. In these circumstances, outside support to maintain the home can be crucial. In addition to the impact on identity, there may be a lack of person–environment fit. Mobility problems in particular can pose serious problems for an older adult, whose home has not been modified accordingly, thereby making daily tasks and access outside the home challenging. These problems can also result in isolation and loneliness. Many older people stress their desire to maintain long-term friendships and social contacts. Community transportation may be not sufficiently flexible or available to help people maintain their preferred social networks. The public infrastructure can also create major barriers to mobility – a lack of public benches, toilets or accessible public transport can have a major impact on the ability of older people to engage in social relationships.

## Promoting independence, choice and control

Despite a multitude of individual conditions and societal forces that threaten the independence of older persons, other opportunities exist to help them regain and sustain choice and control. The next section outlines a number of these key areas.

### Information and advice

Older people, particularly those who are socially isolated, often lack the information and advice that they need to make informed decisions about their lives (JRF 2004b: O'Neil and Dunning 2005; Yardley and Todd 2005).

- Greater information on the services and support that are available locally is needed.
- Advice needs to be tailored to the situation and capabilities of each individual.
- Written information needs to be tailored to those whose first language is not English.
- 'Word of mouth' is often the best medium for getting messages across.
- Older people may need greater support to access and develop computer skills to help them access the information that they require.

## Individually tailored services

Older people represent a wide range of needs and abilities. Consequently, services should be:

- developed and managed by older people themselves;
- focused on supporting existing social networks of family and friends rather than replacing them with new activities and social groups which are not necessarily desirable or appropriate;
- flexible enough to respond to changing health status;
- a means for promoting and maintaining positive outcomes;
- accessible to even the most frail or physically impaired.

For many older people, particularly those who are experiencing a massive transition in their lives, there is a need for greater support and advocacy in helping people build up self-esteem and identify their own solutions.

## Accessible physical environment

Choice and control can be limited simply because of the physical barriers in the environment that can restrict independence. Older people have prioritized the following:

- more public benches and well-maintained pavements;
- more public toilets that feel safe and well maintained;
- better street lighting and greater police presence on the streets to help people feel safe;
- greater access to public and community transport along with comfortable bus stops and station facilities.

More serious challenges again exist for older adults living in rural communities where public transportation is not available. There is a need to develop creative solutions for this population to increase opportunities for community participation and access to services.

### Improved services for older people with high levels of physical and mental frailty

Older people suffering multiple chronic health problems may lack confidence and the ability to utilize services. Not accessing needed services can dramatically compromise one's health and independence. For this vulnerable segment of the older adult population, there is a need to provide:

- improved community transport to and from medical appointments;
- volunteers who can serve as escorts;
- access to affordable domestic help to assist older people with daily tasks related to function;
- home modification and support in maintaining the upkeep.

### Preventative support

Emphasis on treating acute and chronic conditions can often overshadow the need for older individuals to receive preventative care. Older people have prioritized the following:

- access to care for eyes, ears, teeth and feet to maintain independence;
- physiotherapy, occupational therapy and counselling services.

In addition, professionals should be equipped with the skills both to recognize different coping strategies and to help older people consider the options available to them.

## Conclusion

This chapter has outlined a range of factors related to sustaining and threatening independence in later life. It has explored a number of psychological mechanisms that older people adopt to manage the stresses and practical problems associated with physical and mental disability, while also examining some of the external factors which further impede older people's ability to take control over their lives. The wide variation in the ability of older adults to age 'successfully' and adapt to changing health and social status reflects the complexity involved in maintaining independence. Many older adults are highly skilled at accommodating any loss and societal threats, but others may react with lowered self-esteem, a sense of loss of control or by 'giving up'. The challenge is to develop policies, programmes and opportunities that are sensitive to the heterogeneity of older adults while recognizing their overarching need and desire to retain an independent life.

# Reflective questions

1   What are the key factors in life that help one maintain overall independence and control? Is it possible to maintain these in the face of physical, sensory and cognitive disabilities?
2   Why does independence occupy such a central value in Westernized cultures?
3   What factors limit full control over decisions regarding the services or treatments in later life?
4   Consider fears and anxieties one may have with declining health. What strategies would be helpful or adaptive in coping with these changes? What type of support would be acceptable from family, friends or formal care providers?
5   What factors are relevant when considering the balance between independence versus safety?

# Acknowledgements

Acknowledgements go to Phil Rossall and Amy Semple for their input into this chapter.

# References

Albinsson, L. and Strang, P. (2002) A palliative approach to existential issues and death in end-stage dementia care, *Journal of Palliative Care*, 18(3): 168–74.

Almberg, B., Grafström, M. and Winblad, B. (1997) Major strain and coping strategies as reported by family members who care for aged demented relatives, *Journal of Advanced Nursing*. 26(4): 683–91.

Baldock, J. and Hadlow, J. (2002) Housebound older people: the links between identity and use of care services, in *Growing Older Research Findings 4*, Growing Older Programme, ESRC, Sheffield: University of Sheffield.

Baltes, P. B. and Baltes, M. M. (1990) Psychological perspectives on successful aging: the model of selective optimization with compensation, in P. B. Baltes and M. M Baltes (eds) *Successful Ageing: Perspective from the Behavioural Sciences*. Cambridge: Cambridge University Press.

Blanchard-Field, F., Jahnke, H. C. and Camp, C. (1995) Age differences in problem-solving style: the role of emotional salience, *Psychology and Aging*, 10(2): 173–81.

Bowling, A., Banister, D. and Sutton, S. (2002) Adding quality to quantity: older people's views on their quality of life and its enhancement, in *Growing Older Research Findings 7*. Sheffield: Growing Older (GO) Programme, ESRC, University of Sheffield.

Bowman, C., Whistler, J. and Ellerby, M. (2004) A national census of care home residents, *Age and Ageing*, 33: 561–6.

Brown-Wilson, C. (forthcoming PhD) Relationships in nursing homes: a constructivist inquiry. Unpublished PhD thesis, University of Sheffield.

Buckner, L. and Yeandle, S. (2005) *Older Carers in the UK*. London: Carers UK. Available at: http://www.carersuk.org/Policyandpractice/Research/Profileofcaring/ 1207234833/ResearchCaringandolderpeopleNovemeber2005.pdf (Accessed 4 Apr. 2008).

BUPA Care Homes (2006) Census of BUPA care home residents, Continuing Care Conference. June 2006. London, June.

Burnett-Wolle, S. and Godbey, G. (2007) Refining research on older adults' leisure: implications of selection, optimization, and compensation and socioemotional selectivity theories, *Journal of Leisure Research*, 39: 498–513.

Bytheway, B., Ward, R., Holland, C., and Peace, S. (2007) *Too Old: Older People's Accounts of Discrimination, Exclusion and Rejection*. London: Help the Aged.

Carstensen, L. L. (1992) Social and emotional patterns in adulthood: support for socioemotional selectivity theory, *Psychology and Ageing*, 7(3): 331–8.

Cartier, C. (2003) From home to hospital and back again: economic restructuring, end of life, and the gendered problems of place-switching health services, *Social Science and Medicine*, 56: 2289–301.

Cattan, M. (2002) *Supporting Older People to Overcome Social Isolation and Loneliness*. London: Help the Aged.

CDCP (Center for Disease Control and Prevention) (2003) Public health and aging: trends in aging – United States and worldwide, *Morbidity and Mortality Weekly Report*, 52(6): 101–6.

Clarke, A., Seymour, J. E., Welton, M., Sanders, C., and Gott, M. (2006) *Listening to Older People: Opening the Door for Older People to Explore End of Life Issues*. London: Help the Aged.

Davie, G. and Vincent, H. (1998) Religion and old age, *Ageing and Society*, 18: 101–10.

Depp, C. A. and Jeste, D. V. (2006) Definitions and predictors of successful aging: a comprehensive review of larger quantitative studies, *American Journal of Geriatric Psychiatry*, 14(1): 6–20.

Dewar, A. (2003) Boosting strategies: enhancing the self-esteem of individuals with catastrophic illnesses and injuries, *Journal of Psychosocial Nursing & Mental Health Services*, 41(3): 24–32.

Doran, T., Drever, F. and Whitehead, M. (2003) Health of young and elderly informal carers: analysis of UK census data, *British Medical Journal*, 327: 1388.

Fernandez-Ballesteros, R. (2006) GeroPsychology: An applied field for the 21st century, *European Psychologist*, 11(4): 312–23.

Festinger, L. (1954) A theory of social comparison process, *Human Relations*, 7: 117–40.

Folkman, S. and Greer, S. (2000) Promoting psychological well-being in the face of serious illness: when theory, research and practice inform each other, *Psycho-Oncology*, 9: 11–19.

Frieswijk, N., Buunk, B. P., Steverink, N. and Slaets, J. P. (2004) The effect of social comparison information on the life satisfaction of frail older persons, *Psychology and Ageing*, 19(1): 183–90.

Gignac, M. A., Cott, C. and Badley, E. M. (2000) Adaptation to chronic illness and disability and its relationship to perceptions of independence and dependence, *Journal of Gerontology*, 55(6): 362–72.

GMC (General Medical Council) (2002) Withdrawing and withholding life prolonging treatments: good practice in decision making, *Guidance from the Standards Committee of the General Medical Council*. London: GMC.

Godfrey, M. and Denby, T. (2004) *Depression and Older People: Towards Securing Well-being in Later Life*. Bristol: Policy Press.

Goffman, E. (1961) *Asylums*. London: Penguin Books.

Help the Aged (2006) End of life care press briefing, March. London: Help the Aged.

Hopkinson, J. A. and Hallet, C. (2002) Good death? An exploration of newly qualified nurses' understanding of good death, *International Journal of Palliative Nursing*, 8(11): 532–9.

Howarth, G. (1998) Just live for today: living, caring ageing, dying, *Ageing & Society*, 18(6): 673–89.

Howse, K. (2002) The reluctance of older people to accept assistance and support. Unpublished paper. Centre for Policy on Ageing, London.

Jopp, D. and Smith, J. (2006) Resources and life-management strategies as determinants of successful aging: on the protective effect of selection, optimization, and compensation, *Psychology and Ageing*, 21(2): 253–65.

JRF (Joseph Rowntree Foundation) (2004a) *Older People Shaping Policy and Practice*. York: JRF.

JRF (Joseph Rowntree Foundation) (2004b) *Black and Minority Ethnic Older People's Views on Research Findings*. York: JRF.

Koenig, H. G., Larson, D. B. and Larson, S. S. (2001) Religion and coping with serious medical illness, *Annals of Pharmacotherapy*, 35(3): 352–9.

Krause, N. (2002) Church-based social support and health in told age: exploring variations by race, *Journals of Gerontology*, 57(6): S332–47.

Lazarus, R. S. and Folkman, S. (1984) *Stress, Appraisal and Coping*. New York: Springer.

Lynn, J. and Adamson, D. M. (2003) *Living Well to the End of Life: Adapting Health Care to Serious Chronic Illness in Old Age*. Arlington, VA: Rand Health.

MacKinlay, E. (2005) Death and spirituality, in M. Johnson, V. L. Bengtson, P.G. Coleman and T. B. L. Kirkwood (eds) *The Cambridge Book of Age and Ageing*. Cambridge: Cambridge University Press.

McFadden, S. H. (1995) Religion and well-being in aging persons in an aging society, *Journal of Social Issues*, 51: 161–75.

National Statistics (2004). Informal care. Available at: http://www.statistics.gov.uk/cci/nugget_print.asp?ID=925 (accessed 4 Nov. 2008).

O'Neil, A. and Dunning, A. (2005) *Is Information Power? Older People, Information, Advice and Advocacy*. York: Joseph Rowntree Foundation.

Owen, T. (ed.) (2005) *Dying in Older Age*. London: Help the Aged.

Owen, T. and NCHRDF (National Care Home Research and Development Forum) (2006) *My Home Life: Quality of Life in Care Homes*. London: Help the Aged.

Prison Reform Trust (2006) *Old Inside*. Available at: http://www.prisonreformtrust.org.uk/subsection.asp?id=592, (accessed 4 Nov. 2008).

Reed, J., Cook, G., Childs, S. and Hall, A. (2003) *Getting Old is Not for Cowards: Comfortable, Healthy Ageing.* York: Joseph Rowntree Foundation.

Riseborough, M. (2000) *Overlooked and Excluded.* London: Age Concern England.

Rowe, J. and Kahn, R. (1998) *Successful Ageing.* New York: Pantheon Books.

Scharf, T., Phillipson, C., Smith, A. and Kingston, P. (2002) *Growing Older in Social Deprived Areas: Social Exclusion in Later Life.* London: Help the Aged.

Seymour, J. E., Witherspoon, R., Gott, M. et al. (2005) *End of Life Care: Promoting Comfort, Choice and Well-Being among Older People Facing Death.* Bristol: Policy Press.

SPRU (Social Policy Research Unit) (2001) *Informal Care over Time.* York: University of York.

WHO (World Health Organization) (2002) *Active Ageing: A Policy Framework.* Geneva: WHO.

WHO (World Health Organization) (2007) *Global Age-friendly Cities: A Guide.* Geneva: WHO.

Wills, T. A. (1981) Downward comparison principles in social psychology, *Psychological Bulletin*, 90: 245–71.

Wink, P. and Dillon, M. (2001) Religious involvement and health outcomes in late adulthood: findings from a longitudinal study of women and men, in T. G. Plante and A.C. Sherman (eds) *Faith and Health: Psychological Perspectives.* New York: Guilford Press.

Wray. S. (2004) What constitutes agency and empowerment for women in later life? *Sociological Review,* 52(1): 22–38.

Yardley, L. and Todd C. (2005) *Encouraging Positive Attitudes to Falls Prevention in Later Life.* London: Help the Aged.

# 9 Conclusions
## Mima Cattan

## Introduction

In this book we have discussed and explored the wide range of factors associated with older people's mental health and well-being. Most importantly, however, the breadth of subjects covered by the chapters has illustrated the complexity of mental well-being in later life and that no single answer can be provided as to what contributes to older people's mental well-being. As we have seen, older people are 'people' first and 'older' second, and experience the same ups and downs as other age groups do, with one exception: being old frequently means having to deal with a disproportionate set of ongoing, long-term difficulties. Gradual physical decline, loss, fewer resources, and so on can all have an impact on an individual's mental health. HelpAge International has on numerous occasions reported how older people in many countries are neglected or discriminated against, with older women in particular being vulnerable to abuse and loss of rights (HelpAge International 2002). On the other hand, as we have seen, later life can mean release from responsibilities, with more time to spend on oneself, to learn new skills – in other words it can bring a new lease of life. Chapter 2 talks about the 'well-being paradox' whereby, despite the increasing prevalence of health risk factors, there may be a positive relationship between increasing age and subjective well-being. This final chapter pulls together the debates, discussions and conclusions from the preceding chapters, reflects on some of the common themes that run through the chapters, and finally comments on areas needing further attention and the future of the promotion of mental health in later life.

The Introduction discussed what old age means in different cultures, pointing out that older people are not a homogeneous group but vary according to their culture, values, personal make-up, life experiences, and so on. It was acknowledged that 'old age' *per se* is a meaningless term unless it is possible to provide in some way a framework for it. Even with a framework – and in this book the WHO definition was used (WHO 2007) – it has to be accepted that there isn't an exact demarcation of when 'middle age' stops and 'old age' starts. It was therefore accepted that there would be 'variations of old age' throughout the book and also that within the age band of 'old age' there would be variations and differences. An important point was made about the diversity of older people and in what way this needs to be considered in mental health promotion. So, for example, the mental health vulnerability of an older prisoner may be quite different from that of a healthy, well-to-do grandparent.

However, the complexity of the determinants of mental health in later life means that it is not possible to box people neatly into perfect categories of mental well-being, but rather that we need to be responsive to the multitude of factors at play.

This is also reflected in theories of ageing and the way these are linked to theoretical positions in mental health promotion, as discussed in Chapter 3. Many early theories were based on a Western perspective of old age, the assumption that we all respond in the same way to our own ageing process, and that ageing for most people is a highly negative experience. As Chapter 3 showed, it is unlikely or even not desirable that one theory should represent older people's experiences across cultures, societies or even age cohorts. This is obviously an important issue when it comes to mental health promotion practice; do we choose to take a preventive medical or an empowerment approach in our practice, or do we reject a focus on the individual in any form and consider an environmental/ecological approach as the only way forward in promoting the well-being of older people?

Before moving on to the areas identified by older people as important with regards to their mental health, a useful overview and discussion about what is meant by 'mental health' and 'mental well-being' in later life was provided in Chapter 2. It would be easy to rely on the proposed definition by the World Health Organization: 'a state of well-being in which the individual realizes his or her own abilities, can cope with the normal stresses of life, can work productively and fruitfully, and is able to make a contribution to his or her community' (WHO 2004: 11), but does this actually describe fully the meaning of mental health and well-being for an older person? As Chapter 2 showed, we are only just beginning to understand what factors are involved in determining people's mental health and the association between them, and many concepts are still being debated. What is really interesting in this debate is the lack of agreement around the approach to defining mental health. This polarization between a very narrow, individual focused approach and a wider, societal approach is evident in policy, practice and research. These differences have been summarized very neatly by MacDonald (2006) in an overview of mental health promotion theory (see Appendix 1).

## What older people want

Bette Davis is quoted to have said 'Old age is no place for sissies'. It is interesting to ponder what she actually meant by this. Was she simply talking about physical appearance or was she in fact reflecting on the many factors that affect us generally as we age? Would she have worried about becoming isolated and lonely, or about experiencing loss or becoming frail and forgetful? Of course this is purely speculative, and we will never know why she made the comment or if she ever even made the comment in the first place. However, the statement does echo a general perception about old age being tough – somehow older people have to cope with their condition, in other words their 'old age'. And, in our minds 'old age' becomes synonymous with 'mental health problems', which is perhaps why, when older people do have mental health problems it is frequently brushed off as, 'It's your age' – or ignored altogether!

In 'Clare in the community' on page xv we see a typical perspective of old age: an older woman, alone, isolated and lonely who has had the luxury of chatting for two hours with someone – whom she doesn't know and is unlikely to meet again. She does, however, express a need – a need for social contact. We know from research, as the chapters in this book have shown, that social contact is a fundamental need in terms of mental well-being. And we also know from practice and numerous studies that there are a range of interventions such as befriending schemes (or friendship circles as they are increasingly becoming known as) providing such support, which are highly valued by older people (see, for example, Dean and Goodlad 1998; Cattan et al. 2009). But of course, as we've seen, this is not the only expression of a mental health need, or of mental health promotion. Interestingly, the woman mistaken for Mrs Cole in the cartoon is actually supplied with a whole list of services and activities that would provide interest and content to her life as well as reassurance and security, all factors that could be said would contribute to her mental well-being.

The authors in Chapter 4 started by saying that there was a gloominess about mental health in future cohorts of older people, but went on to show how population- or community-level strategies based on policy and practice designed to maximize social inclusion are likely to be effective in improving and maintaining older people's mental health. Chapters 5 to 8 echo these messages, with three rather serious themes relating to mental health in older people running through the four chapters: discrimination because of age (ageism) and the stigma of being old; the need for relationships; and the right to dignity. In some ways you could argue that the themes all refer to older people's human rights, reflecting some of the main priorities listed by the recently launched Global Movement on Mental Health (Patel et al. 2008). These themes will now be explored in more detail in relation to current knowledge and practice and the future of mental health promotion.

## Discrimination because of age and the stigma of being old

Age discrimination is increasingly being legislated against in many countries. However, most such legislation refers to discrimination in employment, for example, the amendment to the Employment Equality (Age) Regulations 2006 that came into force in the UK in April 2008 (Employment Equality 2008), rather than to age discrimination *per se*. Age discrimination can take a variety of forms, from the refusal of services to being ignored by others. Finding that there is an upper age limit for services or goods, being forced off the pavement into the street by others despite obvious mobility difficulties or being talked about as if you're not present are common occurrences that older people have to endure and strongly resent. As far back as the eighteenth century John Wesley, one of the founders of the Methodist Church suggested a 'cure' for old age – demonstrating that old age has for quite some time been something to be avoided for as long as possible, ignored or poked fun at. The stigma of old age is reflected in the 'anti-ageing' movement, where pharmaceutical companies and quacks join forces to appeal to our desires to remain young.

Anti-wrinkle creams, hair dyes and face lifts tempt us to deny or at least put off old age. Several studies have shown (see, for example, Hurd Clark and Griffin 2008; Lund and Engelsrud 2008) that ageism doesn't just stem from 'others' against older people, but that older people frequently reinforce negative stereotypes of old age and maintain ageism and injustice against other older people.

According to the Social Exclusion Unit (SEU), negative attitudes towards age can be compounded by discrimination on the grounds of race, disability, sexual identity, gender or religion (SEU 2006). However, importantly, because everyone can potentially experience prejudice as a consequence of age, ageism is the most common form of discrimination. One of the consequences of ageism and the stigma of old age can be social isolation, which in turn (see Chapter 6) is associated with loneliness and mental health problems. Of course, there are several other factors that contribute to loneliness and social isolation, but at least stigma, prejudice and ageism are issues that can be tackled through mental health promotion. The SEU proposes a multifaceted approach to empower older people and improve their quality of life. This approach, which is intended to improve participation and prevention, includes: advocacy and specialist advice, transport, social activities, health, social care, housing, safety and environment, finance and benefits, information, life-long learning and volunteering (SEU 2006: 9). If we consider the themes running through this book, it would seem that most of these interlinked elements apply in mental health promotion as well. The main message here is that if we are to tackle ageism, stigma and discrimination against older people it is not sufficient to address just one of these areas in isolation, they must all be dealt with. Of course, 'we have to start somewhere' and if that means, for example, eradicating institutional ageism and discrimination then that in itself may lead to further cultural shifts in other areas.

## The right to dignity

According to the *Oxford English Dictionary* (2005) 'dignity' is 'the state of being worthy of respect', 'a calm or serious manner' or 'a sense of pride in yourself'. It is interesting to consider that, on the one hand, it is about individuals' perceptions of themselves – their self-esteem while, on the other hand, it is about other people's judgement of the individual – whether they are worthy of respect. Perhaps it is this tension that links mental health to 'the right to dignity', in other words your own perception of you versus how others view you. There is a huge volume of literature showing that older people want to feel valued, to have a continued role in life, to be able to continue contributing to society and to have a sense of worth. Over and over again it has been shown that there is a strong association between losing a role in life, not feeling valued or respected for what you can offer, being patronized and ignored and serious mental health problems in later life. So why does ageism persist? Looking at the other aspect of dignity, that of 'being worthy of respect' we might start seeing the dichotomy and the answer. As we have already discussed above, if ageism persists, then others who are younger are likely to view older people as not being worthy of respect.

Ronald Blythe in his sombre reflection on old age in *The View in Winter* (Blythe 1981) suggests that the 'problem' of old age is that people are afraid of the stereotype of old age, which doesn't necessarily reflect the reality of older people's lives. As Blythe (1981: 45) states: 'Old age is full of life and full of death. It is a tolerable achievement and it is a disaster. It transcends desire and it taunts it. It is long enough and it is far from being long enough.' And so the judgement about whether or not older people are worthy of respect frequently becomes based on the negative aspects of ageing, such as physical appearance, rather than on the positives of experience and knowledge. Of course this is an enormous generalization and there are plenty of instances where the contrary is true. However, we can't get away from the fact that many older people feel they no longer belong in the social and physical environment around them, not because they are distancing themselves from their surroundings but because they are being rejected by others who are younger. Where does that leave mental health promotion? Interestingly, there have been a number of policy initiatives intended to address issues around dignity, fairness and independency. The NHS Plan, for example, recognizes that service providers frequently fail to view older people as individuals with equal needs for dignity and privacy, and sets out a four-point programme to address this: standards of care should be assured, access to services should be extended; independence should be promoted, and fairness in funding should be assured (DH 2007). This is quite an ambitious programme but one where mental health promotion could have an impact by, for example, developing local strategies in health and social care institutions to ensure that the dignity, privacy and autonomy of older people are respected. Importantly, the emphasis in the programme is on recognizing the diverse needs of older people resulting from differences in gender, ethnicity, disability, sexual identity or religion. This is echoed in several other health and social care documents, giving detailed advice on what is meant by 'dignity in care'.

We have to remember that dignity isn't just about experiences in care services. Older people define dignity more widely as continuing to have an identity, a role to play, recognition for what they have done but also for what they currently do, receiving respect as human beings, being allowed autonomy and independence (Dignity and Older Europeans Project 2004). In mental health promotion terms, it could be argued that these needs reflect the four basic needs in Maslow's Hierarchy of Motivational Needs (Maslow 1970) which have to be met before being able to move on to higher levels of need: the 'growth needs'. Therefore, the need for dignity is closely associated with the notion of self-esteem which, as has been shown throughout the book but particularly in Chapters 2 and 8, is fundamental to mental well-being.

Events around natural disasters, such as the tsunami in December 2004 or Hurricane Katrina in 2005, are extreme examples of how older people are not treated with dignity. Studies following these events found that older people's specific needs were not taken into account either during or after the disaster, and were frequently neglected when it came to any form of aid. In the case of Hurricane Katrina evacuation planning not only put older people at the bottom of the list of priorities, but also it ignored the way older people might respond in emergency situations based on life experiences. Following the tsunami the contribution older people could make in emergency situations and the role they played in the livelihood of families were mostly overlooked and they were simply viewed as (less deserving) recipients of assistance (HelpAge International 2005; Bytheway 2007). The evidence also suggests that subsequently older people's mental health needs were not met or even addressed. Although these are extreme events, older people frequently find themselves similarly compromised in other situations. Here it would seem that the only way mental health promotion is going to make any progress is by adopting a combination of empowerment and social change models to enable older people to be treated with dignity.

There is another aspect of 'dignity' and mental health which isn't related to health services or to receiving respect *per se* but more to the notion of having the same basic rights as other members of society. Many such rights are directed by national or even international policy. Studies have shown that there is an association between mental ill health in later life and the number of stressful life events, the experience of financial difficulties and long-standing physical health problems (Evans et al. 2003). At the time of writing, the global financial crisis has led to large increases in essential basic costs, such as fuel, food, housing and heating. Older people have been hit particularly hard. A report by the Institute for Fiscal Studies (Leicester et al. 2008), supported by Age Concern, has shown that because fuel and food are a greater part of pensioners' outgoings proportionately compared to other age groups, pensioners have a significantly higher rate of inflation than non-pensioners. Unsurprisingly, the most affected are the poorest and the very old. In response to the report, Age Concern called on the UK government to respond through changes to the Basic State Pension and Pension Credit and a range of short-term emergency measures to support older people finding themselves in financial difficulties. Although it is too early to judge the full effect of the current financial crisis on older people's mental health, it is quite clear that income and socio-economic status are associated with mental ill health (Evans et al. 2003; Ladin 2008), demonstrating that for mental health promotion to be effective, it has to function on several planes and in collaboration with other groups.

Food and fuel poverty is an example of where external factors beyond most people's control have an impact on their mental health. The important issue here is that although it can impact adversely on any age group, it's the oldest and poorest who are hit the hardest. In addition, their vulnerability to mental health problems is potentially increased as they are also more likely to have long-standing physical health problems and have experienced numerous stressful life events. The challenge for future mental health promotion is to develop both long-term and medium-term strategies, which enable not just micro activities at the individual level but also macro interventions at the societal level. This is also the case with transport, housing and the quality of the external environment, which are often mentioned by older people as barriers to social participation, and over which they feel they have little or no control (Cattan et al. 2003). Although there is very little research on these issues, a few studies suggest that costly or inaccessible transport, inadequate or unsafe housing and unsafe external environments may lead to social isolation, increased mobility problems and associated mental health problems such as depression (Thomson et al.

2001; Cummins et al. 2005; Marsden et al. 2008). Unfortunately, because of the lack of evaluation of actual interventions to improve housing, transport or other environmental factors for older people, mental health promotion does not have an evidence base which could give direction for future activity. This is clearly an area in urgent need of action and research.

## The need for relationships

Chapter 6 proposed that the most basic need we as human beings have from the day we are born is to have satisfying social relationships with others. It's been suggested that this need is so fundamental to our well-being that the lack of such relationships will ultimately lead to serious mental health problems. There are of course differences in our contacts with others. Relationships vary from intimate companionships, partnerships and immediate family to wider social networks of friends and people providing 'resources'. It would seem that older people have different expectations of the different types of relationships, which is not always understood when services are planned. Obviously the needs for the full spectrum of relationships do not remain static and this has been debated at theoretical level through the much criticized disengagement and activity theories (Burbank 1986). Bond et al. (2007) suggest that rather than thinking of relationships as fixed, we should view them as part of the settings and contexts in which they occur.

Relationships are not, of course, always positive and beneficial for older people. In many parts of the world older people are at increasing risk of violence, crime and abuse. This is important when weighing up options for mental health promotion interventions. Civil conflict, increased levels of crime and drugs-related violence, or high levels of HIV/AIDS increase older people's vulnerability to violence and abusive behaviour. Obviously such violations lead to reduced quality of life and increased risk of mental ill health for older people. Elder abuse can occur in any strata of society and in any culture, and it can take the form of physical abuse, psychological abuse, financial abuse, sexual abuse or neglect. Mistreatment of older people frequently takes place within a complex social and interpersonal context where the solutions are unlikely to be simple or straightforward. A recent survey in the UK found that the prevalence of mistreatment increased with declining health (with a higher prevalence among those who suffered from depression or had recently felt lonely), varied by marital status, socio-economic position and sex, with the majority of perpetrators being either partners/spouses or family members (O'Keeffe et al. 2007). Older people who lived alone were more likely to experience financial abuse than other groups. Importantly, although the majority of older people who had experienced mistreatment sought help, only a small proportion ever reached social services.

On the basis of current social trends we can expect to see larger numbers of older people living independently, alone and without close family nearby. Living alone is a potential risk indicator of mental health problems in later life. It is also likely that friendships will therefore serve an increasingly important role in older people's social networks. These friendships will change and evolve depending on the context and the individual's life stage, with no certainty that they will necessarily remain the same over the life course. The emphasis on changing relationships and friendships will vary between cultures and societies depending on living circumstances, kinships and the perceived role of friendships. The implications for mental health promotion are manifold. On a macro level, inequalities and inequities need to be addressed, while meso-level strategies should ensure access to acceptable and appropriate community based activities, and services and the provision of sufficient support for formal and informal carers to prevent neglect of older people. Micro level activities might include friendship support and enabling older people to have a voice in service development.

Loneliness is frequently quoted as a major problem in old age, despite the majority of older people stating that they are not lonely. In fact, the recorded prevalence of loneliness in later life has not changed in the UK over the past 50 years (Victor et al. 2005). However, as Chapter 6 pointed out, this figure may be higher because the stigma of admitting to being lonely could lead to an under-reporting of the experience. Loneliness has a major impact on quality of life, and we know that there is a close association between loneliness and depression. Indeed, the WHO includes the reduction of loneliness among older people as one of its mental health priorities (WHO 2004). When considering interventions, it needs to be remembered that loneliness in later life can be as a result of a recent event, such as the death of a life-long companion, or carried through the life course because of the individual's personal make-up or a series of life events. Recent research has found six risk factors independently associated with loneliness: widowhood; mental health problems; time spent alone; increased perception of loneliness; actual and perceived poor health (Victor et al. 2005). However, these may not be the only factors associated with loneliness. Many older people in today's rapidly changing world find everyday life complicated and difficult to manage, and express fears of not keeping up with or being part of these changes. Currently we know very little about the vulnerability to loneliness or the quality and characteristics of the experience of loneliness in old age.

As we saw in Chapter 6, there is a fairly strong evidence base for interventions that are effective in combating social isolation and loneliness (Cattan et al. 2005) and nurturing social relationships in later life. Although this is helpful, the demographic, economic and social changes taking place globally at the moment will inevitably mean that other types of interventions also need to be developed, implemented and evaluated. Recent technological advances, for example, have led to an increase in telephone befriending (or friendship circles), and Internet-based social support and social activities to enable older people to develop new friendships. Although the evidence base is still not fully understood, qualitative research suggests that such interventions may help older people to re-engage with their external environment, engage in 'ordinary' social exchanges, and gain confidence and self-respect (Cattan et al. 2009). Again, we need to be cautious and not assume that technology will be the panacea of everything and that virtual relationships will replace every day face-to-face contacts. Like other community-based interventions the purpose of the activity has to be clear. So, for example, it would seem that older people use the Internet and email for different purposes; email is used for social contacts while the Internet is used more for general information and entertainment (whiling the time away).

However, very little is currently known about how and for what purpose older people utilize cell phones or other Internet-based resources, such as social networking platforms.

## Final reflections

Although this book has very clearly set out not to focus on older people with mental illness, cognitive impairment or dementia, we cannot ignore these groups completely with respect to mental health promotion, and some examples have been provided throughout the book. After all, many mental health promoting activities are just as relevant for older people with mental illness or dementia, highlighted in a global campaign driven by the *Lancet*, to recognize the importance of mental health (*Lancet.* 2008). Interestingly, the principles and priorities of an initiative originating from Better Government for Older People (BGOP) in the UK, 'Moving Out of the Shadows' (MOOTS), intended to 'harness the voices of older people who experience a range of mental health problems, to inform and influence future policy, practice and experiences' (Bowers et al. 2005: 1) are for most part applicable to all older people. So, for example, the report suggests that services for older people should be based on what works for older people in terms of their mental well-being, by responding positively to their hopes and aspirations, and by providing them choice and control. With regards to mental health promotion, MOOTS states among other things that it should take a broad approach to achieving and sustaining good mental health in later life, which includes learning, housing, leisure, environment and transport, as well as making policy-makers, commissioners, service providers and practitioners aware of mental health and 'active ageing'. It also recognizes the individual level by suggesting the need for advocacy, counselling support and research into what helps older people living alone to combat isolation and loneliness.

Here it is perhaps useful to reflect on some of the European perspectives of older people's mental health and mental health promotion in the future. At the European level, mental health has not been high on the agenda. However, following a European Community consultative Green Paper on mental health in 2005, which gave some recognition to older people:

> An ageing EU-population, with its associated mental health consequences, calls for effective action. Old age brings many stressors that may increase mental ill health, such as decreasing functional capacity and social isolation. Late life-depression and age-related neuro-psychiatric conditions, such as dementia, will increase the burden of mental disorders.
>
> (CEC 2005: 9)

A European Parliament (2006) Resolution was agreed, stating that one of the greatest challenges facing Europe was its ageing population. This has now led to a 'European Pact' for mental health (EU 2008), supported by the WHO, which includes 'older people' as one of its five priority areas. Considering the broad spectrum of initiatives and interventions illustrated and proposed throughout this book, the EU recommendations seem rather bland (EU 2008: 4):

- promote the active participation of older people in community life, including the promotion of their physical activity and educational opportunities;
- develop flexible retirement schemes which allow older people to remain at work longer on a full-time or part-time basis;
- provide measures to promote mental health and well-being among older people receiving care (medical and/or social) in both community and institutional settings;
- take measures to support carers.

The European strategy on mental health is yet to be published. On the basis of the direction given so far it would seem unlikely that it will outline a holistic evidence based approach to mental health promotion.

In conclusion, as we have seen, there are still tensions between mental health promotion, mental ill health prevention and treatment, and what these actually mean for older people. The lack of a strong evidence base for mental health promotion adds to this dilemma. The chapters in this book have demonstrated that mental health promotion with older people is more than simply a few activities in community centres and that more than anything mental health promotion should be focusing on older people's rights to participate as regular citizens in everyday life. In policy terms this means that older people's views and expectations should be acknowledged and should carry the same weight as the views of others. In practice, we need to develop evidence-based mental health promotion to enable this to become a reality. It also means that we need to move away from the simplistic notion of older people as vulnerable and the recipients of well-meaning services. Of course there are vulnerable older people and those who require a range of services, but many older people, particularly future older people, have a very clear idea about what makes them mentally healthy and how this can be achieved. And, finally, by recognizing that older people's mental well-being is the sum of multiple determinants of health, not just 'health' factors, we can start moving towards innovative and imaginative initiatives to promoting mental health and well-being in later life.

# References

Blythe, R. (1981) *The View in Winter: Reflections on Old Age*. Harmondsworth: Penguin Books.

Bond, J., Dittmann-Kohl, F., Westerhof, G. and Peace. S. (2007) Ageing into the future, in J. Bond, S. Peace, F. Dittmann-Kohl and G. Westerhof (eds) *Ageing in Society*. London: Sage Publications.

Bowers, H., Eastman, M., Harris, J. and Macadam, A. (2005) *Moving Out of the Shadows A Report of Mental Health and Wellbeing in Later Life*. Bournemouth: Help and Care Development.

Burbank, P. M. (1986) Psychosocial theories of aging: a critical evaluation, *Ans – Advances in Nursing Science*, 9(1): 73–86.

Bytheway, B. (2007) *The Evacuation of Older People: The Case of Hurricane Katrina*. London: The Royal Geographical Society and Institute of British Geographers, SSRC.

Cattan, M., Kime, N. and Bagnall, A-M. 2009 *Low-level Support for Socially Isolated Older People: An Evaluation of Telephone Befriending*. London: Help the Aged.

Cattan, M., Newell, C., Bond, J. and White, M. (2003) Alleviating social isolation and loneliness among older people, *International Journal of Mental Health Promotion*, 5(3): 20–30.

Cattan, M., White, M., Bond, J. and Learmonth, A. (2005) Preventing social isolation and loneliness among older people: a systematic review of health promotion interventions, *Ageing and Society*, 25(1): 41–67.

CEC (Commission of the European Communities) (2005) *Improving the Mental Health of the Population: Towards a Strategy on Mental Health for the European Union*. Brussels: European Union.

Cummins, S., Stafford, M., Macintyre, S., Marmot, M. and Ellaway, A. (2005) Neighbourhood environment and its association with self rated health: evidence from Scotland and England, *Journal of Epidemiology & Community Health*, 59(3): 207–13.

Dean, J. and Goodlad, R. (1998) *Supporting Community Participation? The Role and Impact of Befriending*. Brighton: Joseph Rowntree Foundation.

DH (Department of Health) (2007) *The NHS Plan: A Plan for Investment, a Plan for Reform*. London: Department of Health.

Dignity and Older Europeans Project (2004) *Dignity and Older Europeans*. Cardiff: Cardiff University.

Employment Equality (2008) *Employment Equality (Age) Regulations 2006 Amendment Regulations 2008*. Available at: http://www.berr.gov.uk/employment/discrimination/age-discrimination/index.html (accessed 15 Sept. 2008).

EU (European Union) (2008) *European Pact for Mental Health and Well-being*. Brussels: EU.

European Parliament (2006) *Improving the Mental Health of the Population – Towards a Strategy on Mental Health for the EU*. P6_TA(2006)0341. Available at: http://www.europarl.europa.eu/ (accessed 15 Sept. 2008).

Evans, O., Singleton, N., Meltzer, H., Stewart, R. and Prince, M. (2003) *The Mental Health of Older People*. London: Office for National Statistics.

HelpAge International (2002) *State of the World's Older People 2002*. London: HelpAge International.

HelpAge International (2005) *The Impact of the Indian Ocean Tsunami on Older People*. London: HelpAge International.

Hurd Clarke, L. and Griffin, M. (2008) Visible and invisible ageing: beauty work as a response to ageing, *Ageing & Society*, 28(5): 653–74.

Ladin, K. (2008) Risk of late-life depression across 10 European Union countries: deconstructing the education effect, *Journal of Ageing and Health*, 20(6): 653–70.

*Lancet* (2008) A movement for global mental health is launched, *Lancet*, 372: 1274.

Leicester, A., O'Dea, C. and Oldfield, Z. (2008) *The Inflation Experience of Older Households*. London: Institute for Fiscal Studies.

Lund, A. and Engelsrud, G. (2008) 'I am not that old': inter-personal experiences of thriving and threats at a senior centre, *Ageing & Society*, 28(5): 675–92.

MacDonald, G. (2006) What is mental health? in M. Cattan and S. Tilford (eds) *Mental Health Promotion: A Lifespan Approach*. Maidenhead: Open University Press, pp. 8–32.

Marsden, G., Jopson, A., Cattan, M. and Woodward, J. (2008) Understanding the older traveller – stop, look and listen! *Working with Older People*, 12(2): 12–15.

Maslow, A. (1970) *Motivation and Personality*, 2nd edn. New York: Harper and Row.

O'Keeffe, M., Hills, A., Doyle, M. et al. (2007) *UK Study of Abuse and Neglect of Older People: Prevalence Survey Report*. London: National Centre for Social Research, Kings College London.

*Oxford English Dictionary* (Pocket) (2005) Oxford: Oxford University Press.

Patel, V., Garrison, P., Jesus Mari, J. et al. (2008) The *Lancet's* series on global mental health: 1 year on, *Lancet*, 372: 1354–7.

SEU (Social Exclusion Unit) (2006) *A Sure Start to Later Life: Ending Inequalities for Older People*. London: Office of the Deputy Prime Minister.

Thomson, H., Petticrew, M. and Morrison, D. (2001) Health effects of housing improvement: systematic review of intervention studies, *British Medical Journal*, 323: 187–90.

Victor, C., Scambler, S. J., Bowling, A. and Bond, J. (2005) The prevalence and risk factors for loneliness in later life: a survey of older people in Great Britain, *Ageing and Society*, 25(3): 357–75.

WHO (World Health Organization) (2004a) *Prevention of Mental Disorders: Effective Interventions and Policy Options. A Report of the World Health Organization*. Geneva Department of Mental Health and Substance Abuse, WHO, in collaboration with the Prevention Research Centre in the Universities of Nijmegen and Maastricht.

WHO (World Health Organization) (2004b) *Promoting Mental Health: Concepts – Emerging Evidence, Practice. A Report of the World Health Organization*. Geneva. Department of Mental Health and Substance Abuse, WHO in collaboration with the Victorian Health Promotion Foundation and the University of Melbourne.

WHO (World Health Organization) (2007) Definition of an older or elderly person. Available at: http://www.who.int/healthinfo/survey/ageingdefnolder/en/index.html (accessed 7 July 2007).

# Appendix 1 Comparison of theories relating to mental health promotion

| | Albee and Ryan Finn | Resilience theories | Antonovsky's sense of coherence theory | Seedhouse's Foundation Theory | Trent, HEA, Tudor, etc. | MacDonald and O'Hara |
|---|---|---|---|---|---|---|
| Mental illness or mental health? | Mental illness | Mental health | Mental health | Mental health | Mental health | Mental health |
| Individualistic or ecological? | Both | Individual | Both | Both | Individual | Both |
| Comprehensive enough to capture complexity of mental health? | Nearly | No | Possibly | Possibly | No | Yes |
| Acknowledges the interaction between different elements of mental health? | Possibly | No | Yes | Possibly | No | Yes |
| Acknowledges the influence of social factors on mental health? | Yes | No | Yes | Yes | No | Yes |
| Acknowledges both promoting and demoting factors? | Yes | No | Yes | No | No | Yes |
| Acknowledges the social construction and variability of 'mental illness' and 'mental health'? | No | No | Yes | No | No | Yes |
| Any empirical support? | Yes | ?? | Yes | No | No | Yes |
| Useful as a planning tool? | Yes | No | Possibly | Possibly | Possibly | Yes |

*Source:* MacDonald, G. (2006) What is mental health? in M. Cattan and S. Tilford (eds), *Mental Health Promotion: A Lifespan Approach*. Maidenhead: Open University Press/McGraw-Hill.

# Appendix 2 Organizations which are involved in mental health promotion policy, campaigning, research or funding of research: some national and international examples

- *Alzheimer's Society* – leads care and research charity for people with dementia, their families and carers (http://www.alzheimers.org.uk/).
- *Befrienders Worldwide* – work collaboratively with the Samaritans to provide emotional support and reduce suicide (http://www.befrienders.org/).
- *Care Services Improvement Partnership National Mental Health in Later Life Programme* (*CSIP*) provides lots of resources to help practitioners in promoting mental well-being in later life (http://www.olderpeoplesmentalhealth.csip.org.uk/).
- *Centre for Suicide Research* investigates the causes, treatment and prevention of suicidal behaviour (http://cebmh.warne.ox.ac.uk/csr/).
- *Joseph Rowntree Foundation* is one of the largest social policy research and development charities in the UK, and seeks to better understand the causes of social difficulties and explore ways of overcoming them (http://www.jrf.org.uk/).
- *Mental Health Foundation* aims to help people of all ages manage their own mental health; it promotes innovative action across the UK; it helps people to do their own research, which informs policy, practice development and campaigns (http://www.mentalhealth.org.uk).
- *Mental Health Foundation for New Zealand* Their website is designed to deliver knowledge in the area of mental health, by providing access to quality information and resources (http://www.mentalhealth.org.nz/).
- *Mental Health Foundation of Australia* is an organization of professionals, sufferers and their families, related organizations and members of the public. It makes recommendations on mental health policy, encourages and initiates mental health research, and works to remove stigma associated with mental ill health (http://www.mentalhealthvic.org.au/).

- *MIND*. Mind is the leading mental health charity in England and Wales, challenging discrimination, influencing policy, campaigning and providing education (http://www.mind.org.uk/).
- *National Institute for Health and Clinical Excellence (NICE)* – Mental well-being and older people. They provide guidance for occupational therapy and physical activity interventions to promote the mental well-being of older people in primary care and residential care (http://www.nice.org.uk/guidance/index.jsp?action=byId&o=11671).
- *National Institute for Mental Health (NIMHE)* is responsible for supporting the implementation of positive change in mental health and mental health services. They are part of the Care Services Improvement Partnership, and their main sponsor is the Department of Health (http://nimhe.csip.org.uk/index.html).
- *Public Health Observatories* – North East is one of nine regional Public Health Observatories in England and is part of the government's strategy for improving health and reducing health inequalities. North East Public Health Observatory (NEPHO) is responsible for mental health (http://www.nepho.org.uk).
- *Samaritans* is a 24-hours-a-day telephone and email service providing emotional support for people experiencing feelings of distress which could lead to suicide (http://www.samaritans.org.uk/).
- *The Suicide Prevention Resource Center (SPRC)* USA provides prevention support, training and resources to assist organizations and individuals to develop suicide prevention programmes and policies to advance the National Strategy for Suicide Prevention (http://www.sprc.org).

# Glossary

**Chronological age**: refers to the years a person has been living.

**Collectivist**: a strong emphasis on social and group norms and a recognition of interdependency within the group

**Convoy model of social relations**: is a unifying conceptual framework, developed by Toni Antonucci, within which to consider attachment and other close relationships across the lifespan, such as older adults' networks of social relationships.

**Cross-sectional study/survey**: a study conducted at one point in time about, for example, the prevalence of a disease.

**Deterministic**: determinism is a philosophical position that human behaviour, cognition, decisions and actions are causally determined by an unbroken chain of past and current events.

**Evidence-based practice**: is a process of planning, implementing and evaluating programmes developed from evaluated models or interventions to address health issues at individual or community level.

**Executive control**: the processes involved in supervising the selection, initiation, execution and termination of tasks in multi-tasking.

**Functional or health age**: refers to the non-linear functional decline over time that occurs during the process of ageing.

**Functionalist theory**: is a structural (macro-) theory which considers society as a whole system, with all parts inter-related and working together to meet the needs of the components of that society. It is sometimes referred to as a 'consensus theory' because it views societal relationships as harmonious rather than in conflict.

**Healthy Living Centres**: a network of community-based centres in the UK promoting health and healthy lifestyles in deprived areas, funded through partnerships between the NHS, the private sector, regional and national grant-making organizations and local capital.

**Hierarchy of evidence**: grades of evidence based on study designs and their susceptibility to bias.

**Ideology**: describes the complex of values and associated beliefs which provide people with meaning in their lives and influence their preference for particular approaches in their work.

**Inequalities**: the unequal, unjust and unfair hierarchical distribution of health and its determinants.

**Interpretivist**: interpretivism is where social reality is understood as a meaningful construction based on subjective understandings rather than on objective understandings.

**Longitudinal study**: a study that involves the repeated investigation or observation of a phenomenon over a period of time.

**Macro-level determinants**: those determinants that impact at social, national or global level.

**Meso-level determinants**: those determinants that impact at family and community level.

**Meta-analysis**: where several randomized controlled trials (RCTs) on a specific topic have used precisely the same methodology, the results can be statistically combined using the technique of meta-analysis to give an overall summary result of significance and effect size. Particularly useful when several studies have been done that are individually too small to give convincing results.

**Micro-level determinants**: those determinants that impact at individual level.

**Positivist**: positivism is a philosophical position which states that objective accounts of the world can be produced and causal patterns and theories tested through scientific method.

**Primary prevention**: prevention of disease or mental disorders in susceptible individuals or populations through (mental) health promotion or specific protection e.g. immunization.

**Quality of life**: a multidimensional construct consisting of factors such as health, housing, income, social networks along with subjective perceptions of these factors together with well-being.

**Randomized controlled trial** (**RCT**): a controlled experimental research design use to test a hypothesis.

**Resilience**: is the positive capacity of people to cope with and adapt to adversity, trauma and stress.

**Salutogenesis**: a theory developed by Antonovsky which focuses on factors that support health and well-being rather than on factors that cause disease.

**Secondary level intervention**: action, e.g. screening, taken to identify and treat the early symptoms of a disease with the aim of stopping or reversing the problem.

**Secondary prevention**: see *secondary level intervention*.

**Social capital**: describes social relationships within societies or communities, consisting of community networks, civic engagement, sense of belonging, norms of cooperation and trust.

**Social exclusion**: is complex and multi-dimensional. It means not being able to access things in life that most people take for granted and being unable to participate in normal relationships and activities.

**Systematic review**: is an appraisal of all available research literature focused on a single question of what works (is effective) for a specific health problem.

**Tertiary level intervention**: refers to measures to reduce and limit the negative impact of a health problem/disease which is not fully treatable.

# Index

# EXCELLENCE IN DEMENTIA CARE
Research into Practice

**Murna Downs and Barbara Bowers (eds)**

*'Dementia care has come of age with this book. It is an impeccably crafted collection of papers from eminent experts on both sides of the Atlantic. The book demonstrates confidence, based on both research evidence and well-grounded good practice, and a solid set of shared values both explicit and implicit. The contributors are refreshingly candid about debates and controversies. This book is authoritative and readable which makes it useful to a wide audience. It will provide knowledge, encouragement and motivation to a hard pressed workforce.'*
Mary Marshall OBE, Emeritus Professor, University of Stirling, Scotland

This landmark textbook draws on the extensive knowledge of researchers, practitioners, and professionals in the care of people with Alzheimer's disease and other dementias. It is informed both by a profound respect for people with dementia and a commitment to including them in decisions about their care and lives. While focusing on care for people with dementia, this core text also addresses the most pressing concerns of families by promoting practices and services that recognise the full humanity of their relative with dementia. In addressing the many complex issues related to offering support to people with dementia and those who care for them, this timely textbook is unique in emphasising strategies for creating sustainable change in practice. The book includes examples from a range of countries, drawn from research, practice wisdom and, most importantly, from the experience of people with dementia and their families.

This key text offers valuable insights about how to:

- Provide competent and compassionate care for people with Alzheimer's Disease and other dementias
- Build systems to provide effective care
- Encourage collaboration among multi disciplinary professionals and users and carers
- Support those caring for people with dementia
- Ensure those with dementia maintain dignity, well-being and meaningful participation in life

*Excellence in Dementia Care* is a vital resource for those working with people with dementia. It provides an accessible yet sophisticated overview of the knowledge, skills and attitudes required to achieve excellence. It is an essential handbook for those responsible for training, education and skills development in dementia care.

**Contents:** *Contributors – Foreword – Preface – Acknowledgements – Introduction – Part 1: Principles and perspectives – Prevalence and projections of dementia – Toward understanding subjective experiences of dementia – Ethnicity and the experience of dementia – A bio-psycho-social approach to dementia – Flexibility and change: the fundamentals for families coping with dementia – Towards a person-centred ethic in dementia care: doing right or being good? – Being minded in dementia: persons and human beings – Part 2: Knowledge and skills for supporting people with dementia – Assessment and dementia – Supporting cognitive abilities – Working with life history – The language of behaviour – Communication and relationships: an inclusive social world – Supporting health and physical well-being – Understanding and alleviating emotional distress – Part 3: Journeys through dementia care – Diagnosis and early support – Living at home – Care of people with dementia in the general hospital – The role of specialist housing in supporting people with dementia – Care homes – End of life care – Grief and bereavement – Part 4: Embedding excellence in dementia care – Involving people with dementia in service development and evaluation – A trained and supported workforce – Attending to relationships in dementia care – Leadership in dementia care – Quality: the perspective of the person with dementia – Reframing dementia: the policy implications of changing concepts – The history and impact of dementia care policy – Index.*

2008   640pp
978-0-335-22375-6 (Paperback)   978-0-335-22374-9 (Hardback)

# THE SOCIAL WORLD OF OLDER PEOPLE

Understanding Loneliness and Social Isolation in Later Life

## Christina Victor, Sasha Scambler and John Bond

Developments to the physical environment, scientific and technological innovation, the reorganisation of work and leisure and the impact of globalization and global capitalism have all influenced the nature of the world in which we now live. Social engagement and relationships, however, remain important at any age and their quality is a key element contributing to the quality of life of older people.

This book provides a detailed account of loneliness and social isolation as experienced by older people living in Britain. The authors consider the incidence and effects of isolation and loneliness, identifying the factors which lead to such experiences and considering potential interventions. They also argue that these feelings are experienced at all stages of the life course and not unique to the social world of older people.

Victor, Scambler and Bond rationalise that this is an important area, as both loneliness and social isolation are negatively associated with both quality and quantity of life – whilst the maintenance of social relationships is seen as a key component of 'successful ageing'.

*The Social World of Older People* is important reading for students of social work, gerontology, community care and social policy as well as being of interest to policy makers and practitioners in these fields.

**Contents:** *Preface and Acknowledgements – Introduction – Loneliness and social isolation: issues of theory and method – Social relations and everyday life – Experiences of loneliness – Social exclusion and social isolation – Rethinking loneliness and social isolation in later life – References – Index.*

2008   232pp
978-0-335-21521-8 (Paperback)   978-0-335-21522-5 (Hardback)